HDL Deficiency and Atherosclerosis

DEVELOPMENTS IN CARDIOVASCULAR MEDICINE

VOLUME 174

HDL Deficiency and Atherosclerosis

edited by

G. ASSMANN

Institut für Arterioskleroseforschung
Westfalische Wilhelms-Universität
Münster
Germany

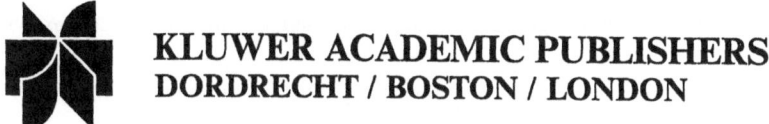

KLUWER ACADEMIC PUBLISHERS
DORDRECHT / BOSTON / LONDON

Distributors

for the United States and Canada: Kluwer Academic Publishers, PO Box 358, Accord Station, Hingham, MA 02018-0358, USA

for all other countries: Kluwer Academic Publishers Group, Distribution Center, PO Box 322, 3300 AH Dordrecht, The Netherlands

A catalogue record for this book is available from the British Library.

ISBN-13: 978-94-011-6587-7   e-ISBN-13: 978-94-011-6585-3
DOI: 10.1007/978-94-011-6585-3

Library of Congress Cataloging-in-Publication Data

HDL deficiency and atherosclerosis / edited by G. Assmann.
    p. cm. – (Developments in cardiovascular medicine ; 174)
    Includes bibliographical references and index.
    ISBN-13: 978-94-011-6587-7
    1. Atherosclerosis–Molecular aspects.   2. High density lipoproteins–
Metabolism–Disorders.   3. Hypolipoproteinemia.   I. Assmann, G. (Gerd)
II. Series: Developments in cardiovascular medicine ; v. 174.
    [DNLM: 1. Lipoproteins, HDL Cholesterol–deficiency.   2. Lipoproteins, HDL
Cholesterol–metabolism.   3. Atherosclerosis–metabolism.   W1 DE997VME v.174
1995 / QU 95 H431 1995]
RC692.H38   1995
616.1'36–dc20
DNLM/DLC
for Library of Congress   95-31820
                                         CIP

Contents

List of Contributors

J. ALBERS
Division of Metabolism, Endocrinology
  and Nutrition
Department of Medicine
University of Washington
Seattle
WA 98195
USA

D. APPLEBAUM-BOWDEN
National Institutes of Health
National Heart, Lung and Blood
  Institute
Molecular Diseases Branch
Bldg.10, Room 7N115
10 Center Dr. MSC 1666
Bethesda
MD 20892-1666
USA

G. ASSMANN
Institut für Arterioskleroseforschung
Westfälische Wilhelms-Universität
Domagkstr. 3
D-48149 Münster
Germany

H.B. BREWER Jr
National Institutes of Health
National Heart, Lung and Blood
  Institute
Molecular Diseases Branch
Bldg.10, Room 7N115
10 Center Dr. MSC 1666
Bethesda
MD 20892-1666
USA

B.G. BROWN
Cardiology RG-22
University of Washington
Health Science Bldg. A-509
Seattle
WA 98195
USA

D.R. BROWN
National Institutes of Health
National Heart, Lung and Blood
  Institute
Molecular Diseases Branch
Bldg.10, Room 7N115
10 Center Dr. MSC 1666
Bethesda
MD 20892-1666
USA

P. BRYSCH
Institut für Arterioskleroseforschung
Westfälische Wilhelms-Universität
Domagkstr. 3
D-48149 Münster
Germany

G.R. CASTRO
SERLIA & U. INSERM 325
Institut Pasteur
1 rue due Professeur Calmette
F-59019 Lille Cedex
France

A. CHAIT
Division of Metabolism, Endocrinology
  and Nutrition
Department of Medicine
University of Washington
Seattle
WA 98195
USA

M. CHEUNG
Division of Metabolism, Endocrinology
  and Nutrition
Department of Medicine
University of Washington
Seattle
WA 98195
USA

C. De GETEIRE
SERLIA & U. INSERM 325
Institut Pasteur
1 rue due Professeur Calmette
F-59019 Lille Cedex
France

B. DELFY
SERLIA & U. INSERM 325
Institut Pasteur
1 rue due Professeur Calmette
F-59019 Lille Cedex
France

T. ENGEL
Institut für Arterioskleroseforschung
Westfälische Wilhelms-Universität
Domagkstr. 3
D-48149 Münster
Germany

L.D. FISHER
Department of Biostatistcs
University of Washington
School of Public Health and Community
   Medicine
Seattle
WA 98195
USA

M. FOBKER
Institut für Arterioskleroseforschung
Westfälische Wilhelms-Universität
Domagkstr. 3
D-48149 Münster
Germany

J.C. FRUCHART
SERLIA & U. INSERM 325
Institut Pasteur
1 rue due Professeur Calmette
59019 Lille Cedex
France

H. FUNKE
Institut fur Klinische Chemie und
   Laboratoriumsmedizin
Zentrallaboratorium
Westfälische Wilhelms-Universität
Albert-Schweitzer-Str 33
D-48149 Münster
Germany

J.M. HOEG
National Institutes of Health
National Heart, Lung and Blood
   Institute
Molecular Diseases Branch
Bldg.10, Room 7N115
10 Center Dr. MSC 1666
Bethesda
MD 20892-1666
USA

Y. HUANG
Institut für Arterioskleroseforschung an
   der Universität Munster
Domagkstrasse 3
D-48149 Münster
Germany

V.S. KASHYAP
National Institutes of Health
National Heart, Lung and Blood
   Institute
Molecular Diseases Branch
Bldg.10, Room 7N115
10 Center Dr. MSC 1666
Bethesda
MD 20892-1666
USA

N. MAEDA
Department of Pathology
University of North Carolina at Chapel
   Hill
Chapel Hill
NC 27599-7525
USA

V.M.G. MAHER
Division of Metabolism, Endocrinology
   and Nutrition
Department of Medicine
University of Washington
Seattle
WA 98195
USA

R.W. MAHLEY
Gladstone Institute of Cardiovascular
   Disease
PO Box 419100
San Francisco
CA 94141-9100
USA

M. RAABE
Institut für Arterioskleroseforschung
Westfälische Wilhelms-Universität
Domagkstr. 3
D-48149 Münster
Germany

R.L. REDDICK
Department of Pathology
University of North Carolina at Chapel
  Hill
Chapel Hill
NC 27599-7525
USA

S. RUST
Institut für Klinische Chemie und
  Laboratoriumsmedizin
Zentrallaboratorium
Westfälische Wilhelms-Universität
Albert-Schweitzer-Str 33
D-48149 Münster
Germany

S. SANTAMARINA-FOJO
National Institutes of Health
National Heart, Lung and Blood
  Institute
Molecular Diseases Branch
Bldg.10, Room 7N115
10 Center Dr. MSC 1666
Bethesda
MD 20892-1666
USA

S. SCHEEK
Institut für Arterioskleroseforschung
Westfälische Wilhelms-Universität
Domagkstr. 3
D-48149 Münster
Germany

U. SEEDORF
Institut für Arterioskleroseforschung
Westfälische Wilhelms-Universität
Domagkstr. 3
D-48149 Münster
Germany

T SZYPERSKI
Swiss Institute of Technology
ETH-Honggerberg
Zurich
Switzerland

A. VON ECKARDSTEIN
Institut fur Klinische Chemie und
  Laboratoriumsmedizin
Zentrallaboratorium
Westfälische Wilhelms-Universität
Albert-Schweitzer-Str 33
D-48149 Münster
Germany

H. WIEBUSCH
Institut fur Klinische Chemie und
  Laboratoriumsmedizin
Zentrallaboratorium
Westfälische Wilhelms-Universität
Albert-Schweitzer-Str 33
D-48149 Münster
Germany

K. WÜTHRICH
Swiss Institute of Technology
ETH-Honggerberg
Zurich
Switzerland

S.H. ZHANG
Department of Pathology
University of North Carolina at Chapel
  Hill
Chapel Hill
NC 27599-7525
USA

XUE-QIAO ZHAO
Cardiology RG-22
University of Washington
Health Science Bldg. A-509
Seattle
WA 98195
USA

Preface

The tandem pace of medical knowledge and prevention of ischaemic heart disease over the past 50 years is testimony to the effectiveness of a combination of massive scientific research, continuous transfer of the results to medical practice, community actions and population awareness. The death rate from coronary heart disease in the United States rose 20% from 1950 to 1963, when a dramatic and steady downward inflection began, arriving today at a rate over 50% lower. Numerous factors have contributed to this success. By 1950 lipoproteins had just been discovered, but a decade later a great surge in research had focussed upon plasma cholesterol and lipoprotein concentrations as major predictors of risk. Today, a continuing expansion and sophistication of that research has removed all doubt about the significance of particular patterns. The pathway to ideal prophylaxis, however, particularly for risks associated with inherited lipoprotein disorders, still awaits the untangling of great amounts of new information that continue to rise from application of molecular technology.

This volume deals with many of the contemporary puzzles. One theme revolves about the high density lipoproteins. For twenty years the HDL have been considered a defence against the caprices of the LDL, now believed to be particularly villainous after oxidation. Increasing discovery of genetically-determined HDL deficiency disorders raises questions, however, about the roles of the several A apoproteins in HDL and various lipid transfer factors in the transfer of cholesterol from cells to the liver by HDL. In studies in mice in which genes for apoproteins have been deleted or genes for human apoproteins have been transfected it has been demonstrated that apoprotein A-1 may counteract the hyperlipidaemia and atherosclerosis found in apo-E deficient mice. The interesting update provided here of experiments in man and animals on transfer of genes for the LDL receptor, A or E apoproteins and for hepatic lipase, indicate that we are nearing the edge of the future for treating severely heightened risk factors due to genetic lipoprotein defects.

Description is also included in this volume of how different isomers 3 and 4 of apo E affect nervous tissues in vitro, the apo E-4 isomer having recently been discovered to be associated with Alzheimer's disease. One can be assured that such deviation is a sign of health in a field of research that is now spilling over to adjacent areas of medical importance. Understanding lipoproteins has not lost its central purpose in relation to cardiovacular disease. The lookout for more effective universal preventives of premature atherosclerosis remains bright.

Donald S. Fredrickson

1

Molecular genetics approach to lipoprotein metabolism disorders

H. FUNKE, H. WIEBUSCH, S. RUST and G. ASSMANN

INTRODUCTION

In past decades epidemiological studies have identified several risk factors for early-onset coronary artery disease (CAD[1-3]). Among these factors disorders of lipoprotein metabolism have a leading role. The PROspective CArdiovascular Münster (PROCAM) study, carried out in the northwest of Germany, has demonstrated that among all single-parameter biochemical markers the concentration of plasma lipids has the highest predictive value.

There are different degrees of association between the incidence of myocardial infarctions and the three main forms of lipoprotein metabolism disorders, hypercholesterolaemia, hypertriglyceridaemia and high density lipoprotein (HDL) reduction. In addition, it is not unusual that these disorders occur in combination. Yet another complicating factor is that these easy-to-determine variations in plasma lipids do not have a common aetiological determinant. This can be illustrated by the fact that, e.g., a hypercholesterolaemia can in one case be caused largely by dietary mistakes, whereas in another case the only aetiological factor is an inherited gene defect.

Even though the results from the PROCAM study and other prospective studies have clearly demonstrated a close link between lipoprotein metabolism and the risk of developing CAD, this knowledge is often difficult to translate into individual risk and the correct strategy for treatment. One possibility to improve risk prediction for the individual may be the breakdown of risk factors into aetiologically distinct entities. The formation of phenotype subgroups and a differentiated risk assessment might thus be possible based on underlying genetic defects.

GENETICALLY DETERMINED LIPOPROTEIN METABOLISM DISORDERS

Biochemical and genetic analyses in families of myocardial infarction patients have led to the identification of numerous gene defects that influence lipoprotein metabolism. These defects also occur more frequently in CAD families than in the general population. Primarily, defects in the LDL receptor (LDL-R) gene, in the genes for apolipoproteins (apo) B, E, A-I, C-II and (a) and in lipoprotein lipase are involved. Clinical phenotypes can be the consequence of defects that influence gene regulation as well as of those mutations that alter the structure of the encoded protein. Today we know that the vast majority of genetically determined lipoprotein metabolism disorders (e.g. familial forms of hypercholesterolaemias) is caused by manifold defects at different gene loci. Currently more than 200 mutations in four different genes (LDL-receptor, apolipoproteins B, E, and [a]) are known to influence plasma cholesterol concentration. The extent of the deviation from normal is a function of the gene involved, and also of the specific mutation.

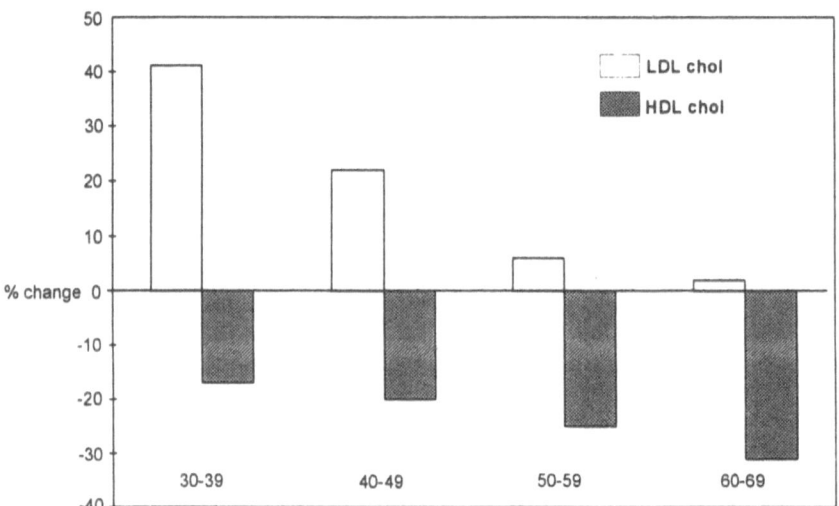

Fig. 1   Relation between age and different CAD risk factors. The graph shows the differences in serum concentrations of LDL-cholesterol and HDL-cholesterol between a population of myocardial infarction survivors and a control group from the general population separated into age decades

Autosomal dominant or codominant forms of lipoprotein metabolism disorders are much less frequent than those with a complex aetiology. The latter often result from a multitude of interactions among different genetic components, and of these components with environmental factors. They are therefore termed multifactorial and polygen in nature. This latter group of lipid metabolism disorders is most frequently seen among survivors of myocardial infarction (MI). The same patients often also have elevated blood pressure and plasma glucose or insulin levels. Interestingly, in the younger MI patient elevated levels of LDL-cholesterol or Lp(a) are frequently observed, while at a higher age HDL-cholesterol reduction, often coexisting with hypertriclyceridaemia, is the predominant finding.

Results from epidemiological investigations in Germany (PROCAM study) showed that a subgroup of the population with extraordinarily elevated CAD risk can be identified. This group includes males aged 40–65 years at study, and is characterized by an elevated LDL-cholesterol/HDL-cholesterol ratio (>5) (Fig.2)[3]. A genetic component in this type of dyslipidaemia relates to the positive family history for MI which is often reported by affected individuals.

Identification of genetic defects in lipoprotein metabolism

General strategies

In general, two different strategies have been used in the identification of genetic defects underlying lipoprotein metabolism disorders[4]. One is the top-down approach, which starts with a detailed characterization of the phenotype and eventually leads to the formulation of a candidate gene. The exact defect is subsequently determined by DNA sequencing and a causal relationship between the genotype and the phenotype is ascertained by biochemical and statistical procedures. The alternative strategy, the bottom-up approach, starts with a gene locus, where structural variance is analysed, and then establishes the phenotypic impact of the observed mutations. This procedure can be used with randomly chosen gene loci and with candidate genes (Fig. 3). Associations of such identified mutations with biochemical or clinical phenotypes have been more stable when the DNA change was predictive also of (structural) changes in the candidate-gene encoded protein. This observation, and the high allelicity of gene defects, explains in part why

3

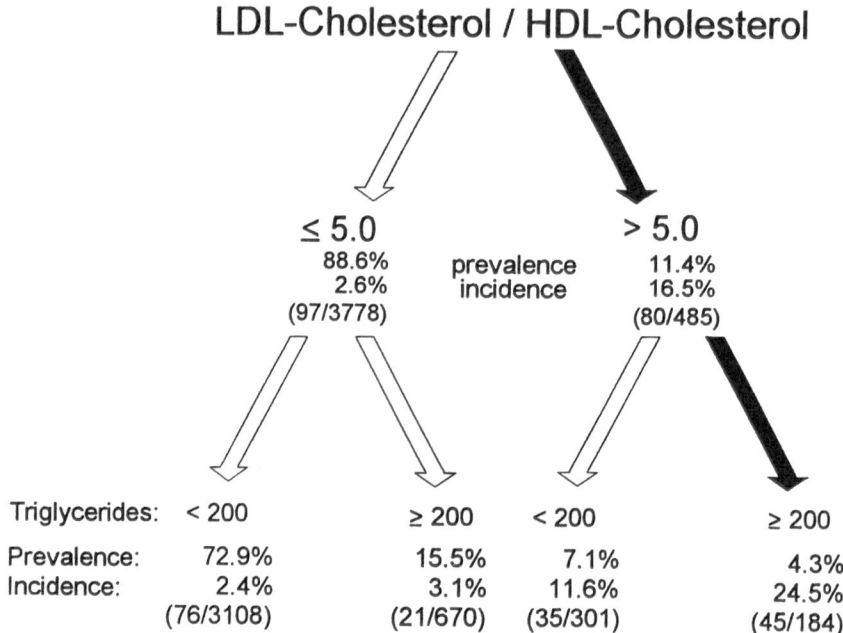

Fig. 2 Role of triglycerides, LDL-cholesterol and HDL-cholesterol for CHD incidence[3]

associations of restriction fragment length polymorphisms (RFLP), which are often located in functionally irrelevant areas of the genome, have not led to the initially expected success in disease prediction. Another reason is the high degree of linkage disequilibrium that often exists between marker mutation and disease mutation, even when they are located within short physical distances of each other.

Reasons for the still low number of lipoprotein metabolism disorders for which the structural basis is known are manifold. The high number of variables influencing the phenotypic parameters used in the description of these disorders largely reduces the efficacy of classical linkage analysis in discovering a disease-specific locus. In many instances the manifestation of a phenotype requires, in addition to a gene mutation, unfavourable external conditions. Moreover, in many lipoprotein anomalies the presence of a familial disease may be mimicked by the high prevalence of an abnormal phenotype, which is defined by a quantitative parameter beyond a threshold value. Another reason lies in the interactions which various components of lipoprotein metabolism

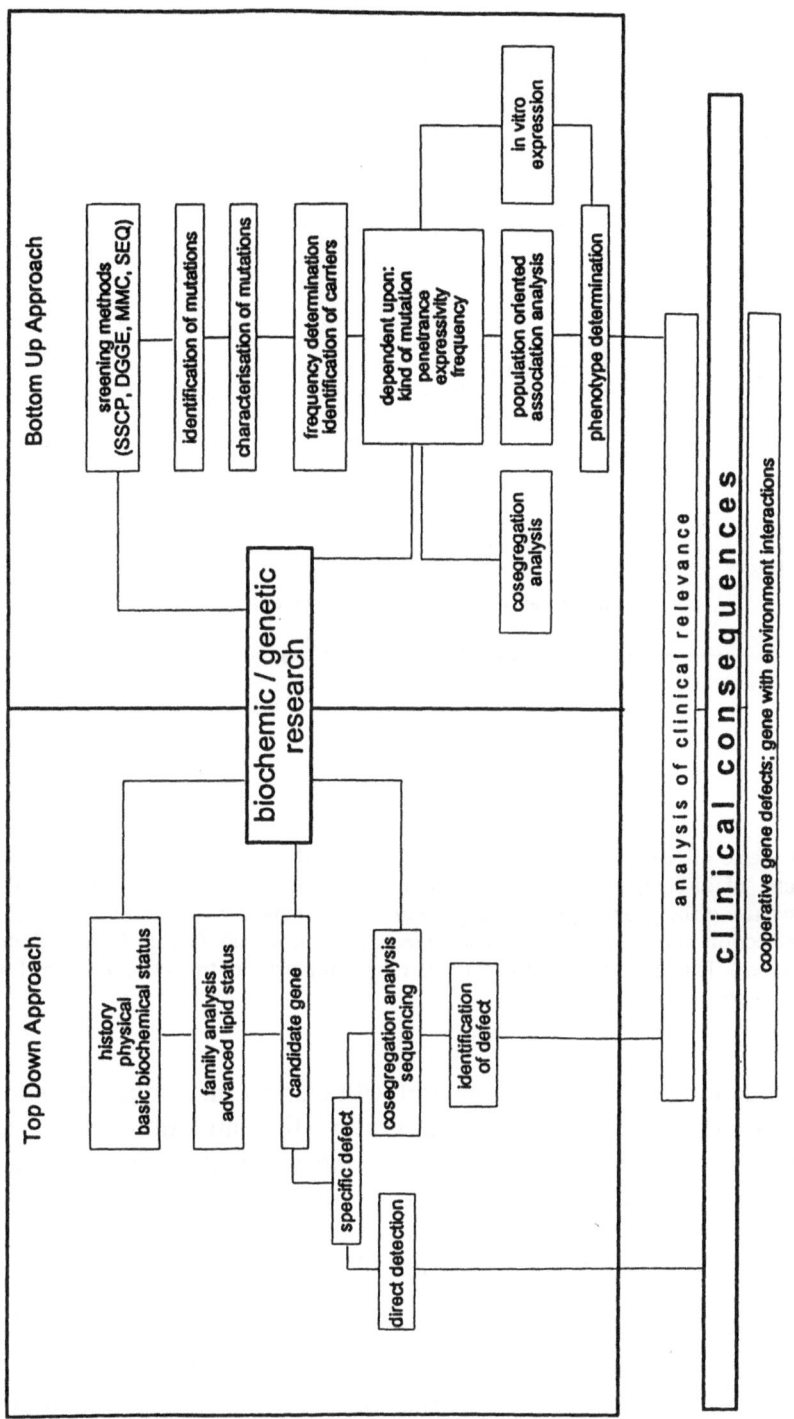

Fig. 3 Strategies for the identification of genetic defects causing lipoprotein metabolism disorders

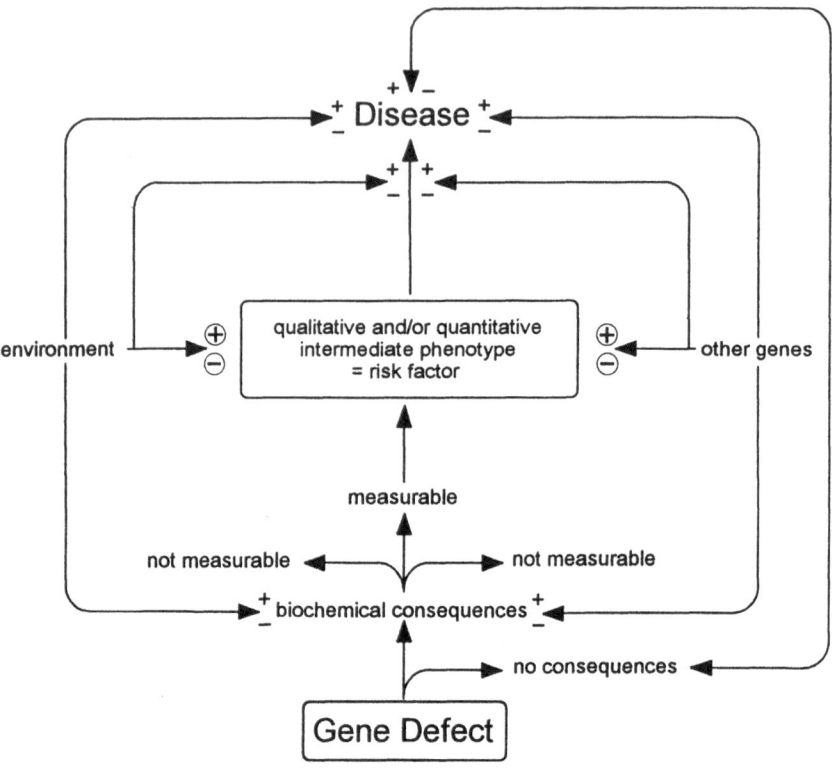

Fig. 4 Role of risk factors in complex genetic disorders. Practical (cost, late-onset character of disease) and ethical reasons made it impossible to carry out family analyses using the phenotype coronary stenosis. Consequently genetic analysis deals with detection and evaluation of basic defects leading to risk factors (intermediate phenotypes). The figure is meant to illustrate the complexity of this task; + stands for positive, – for negative effect

frequently have with one another and with distinct metabolic pathways (Fig. 4). It is also a frequent observation that mutations not only influence the immediate metabolism of the products encoded by the affected gene but can also lead to numerous abnormalities in distantly related pathways. Consequently, it is not easy to discriminate between direct and related effects of a mutation. This illustrates the difficulties of a symptom-related strategy such as the top-down approach in identifying candidate genes.

The opposite strategy, which starts with the identification of mutations and only then looks for their phenotypic consequences (bottom-up approach), is usually successful in determining the consequences of a specific mutation. This can be done using statistical procedures. Although, in principle, this procedure can be used with both anonymous DNA sequence and candidate genes, in practice it is largely reduced to the classical candidate gene approach. While many genes harbour mutations which affect the structure and/or concentration of the encoded protein at a high frequency (e.g. lipoprotein lipase [LPL], hepatic lipase [HPL], others are only rarely affected by mutations (e.g. apolipoprotein [apo] A-I, lecithin: cholesterol acyltransferase [LCAT]). Therefore, before mutation screening is performed, mutation carriers need to be enriched in the screening population. This is usually done based on biochemical knowledge.

Strategies in individual medicine

A dominant pattern of inheritance of a specific lipoprotein phenotype is indicative of the disorder's genetic foundation and allows its separation from polygenic and complex forms of dyslipoproteinaemia showing the same phenotype. As a consequence of the high number of lipoprotein anomalies which have a genetic basis the diagnosis of lipoprotein metabolism disorders should, whenever possible, involve the family of the proband. Even though clinical disease management is not currently based on genetic variation family analyses are essential for early identification of individuals at risk.

The differentiation of a specific phenotype, such as excessive elevation of LDL-cholesterol, into familial and sporadic forms will enable us to test if distinct causes of the same phenotype respond to therapy differently. If useful, further subdifferentiation can be based on single genetic defects (see below).

Using carrier frequencies of 1:500 and 1:700, figures which have been suggested for familial hypercholesterolaemia (FH)[5] and familial defective apoB-100 (FDB)[6] (Table 1), respectively, and assuming that the vast majority of affected individuals have serum LDL-cholesterol concentrations above the 97th percentile of the age- and sex-matched population-distribution curve this results in a prevalence of 7% and 5%, respectively, among individuals with excessive hypercholesterolaemia. While in the LDL-receptor gene more than 150 defective alleles have been identified[7], only a few mutations in apoB are associated with hypercholesterolaemia[8,9]. Among these the mutation causing FDB (Arg3500-

Table 1   Genetic defects affecting total plasma cholesterol levels

Affected gene	Mutation(s)	Carrier frequencies	Changes in total plasma cholesterol
LDL-receptor	Multiple[a]	1:500	50–400% increase[b]
Apolipoprotein B	Arg3500GIn	1:700	25–125% increase[c]
	Arg3531Cys	Unknown	35% increase
	Truncations	Unknown	30–100% decrease[d]
	Other mutations[e]	Probably frequent	Unknown
Apolipoprotein E	Cys112Arg	1:5	0–15% increase[f]
	Arg158Cys	1:7	0–25% decrease[f]
	Rare mutations[g]	Unknown	Variable
Lipoprotein (a)	Multiple	High	Variable[h]

[a] More than 150 different defects have been identified which result in a reduction of cellular cholesterol uptake and an increase in serum cholesterol. Only in founder populations and in some ethnic groups have single mutations been found at a higher frequency.

[b] In heterozygotes the elevation is 50–150%; in homozygotes it is 200–400%.

[c] The extent of serum cholesterol elevation is not different between heterozygote and homozygote carriers.

[d] Heterozygosity causes approximately half normal concentrations and may decrease CAD risk; homozygoisty causes familial hypobetalipoproteinaemia and symptoms similar to abetalipoproteinaemia.

[e] Sequence analysis has shown the presence of multiple deviations from the wild-type sequence. Phenotypic consequences of most of these mutations are currently unknown.

[f] There is a large interindividual variance in phenotype change. The numbers given relate to homozygosity.

[g] Some mutations do not affect serum lipid concentrations; others contribute to dominant type III hyperlipidaemia.

[h] Observed effects depend on the classification system used.

GIn) is the best characterized. There is, however, still an enormous potential for the identification of additional mutations in both genes which could also expand their roles in the formation of hypercolesterolaemia. In the case of the LDL-receptor gene most sequencing analysis has been done in individuals with both a clearly identifiable familial form of hypercholesterolaemia and reduced ligand binding to the receptor. This leaves mutations with mild phenotypic consequences still to be discovered. In the case of apoB it is presumably the enormous size of its gene that has delayed our understanding of genotype–phenotype

Table 2 Genetic defects affecting plasma HDL-cholesterol levels

Affected gene	Mutation(s)	Carrier frequencies	Changes in plasma HDL-cholesterol
Apolipoprotein A-I (apoA-I)	Missense mutations Other mutations [c]	1:1000[a] Very rare	0–95% decrease[b] HDL not measurable
Lecithin:cholesterol acyltransferase (LCAT)	a,b-type[d] (familial LCAT deficiency) a-type[d] (fish-eye disease)	Very rare Very rare	HDL not measurable HDL not measurable
Lipoprotein lipase (LPL)	Asp9Asn Asn291Ser Ser447End Multiple rare mutations[e]	1:35 1:20 1:5 ~1:300[f]	Unknown 5–15% decrease 5–15% increase 0–80% decrease
Cholesterol ester transfer protein (CETP)	Ile 405Val Multiple rare mutations	50–70%[g] Unknown	10% increase[h] Up to 500% increase
Lysosomal acid lipase (LAL)	Frequent missense mutations Multiple rare mutations	>1:20 Unknown	Not known 10–70% reduction
Others	Unknown	~1:6[i]	Variable

[a] Estimation based on experimentally determined frequency of 1:2000 for electrically non-neutral mutations.

[b] Some mutations do not affect HDL-cholesterol, others have a large effect (e.g. Pro165Arg, Arg173Cys).

[c] Nonsense mutations, deletions, insertions, inversions, etc.

[d] The a,b-type is characterized by the complete absence of LCAT activity from plasma and is clinically characterized by a close association with renal failure; the a-type is characterized by the selective loss of LCAT activity using HDL particles as substrate. The only clinical symptom is corneal clouding. Neither type is associated with CAD. Recently LCAT deficiency with residual LCAT activity and mild clinical symptoms has been described.

[e] Homozygosity causes familial chylomicronaemia (type I hyperlipidaemia, in some cases type V hyperlipidaemia). It is accompanied by HDL-deficiency. Heterozygosity causes only small effects; they can be aggravated by dietary mistakes or the presence of other gene defects.

[f] Rough estimation based on sequencing data in hypertriglyceridaemics.

[g] Different carrier frequencies in ethnically distinct populations.

[h] Effect of homozygosity. Same effect in all populations.

[i] Based on the 35 mg/dl risk threshold value, which is the 17th percentile of the frequency distribution curve in Westfalia.

relations. Comparison of seven published sequences for the apoB gene or cDNA has identified 60 differences, many of which were predictive for changes in the encoded protein's amino acid sequence[10]. This demonstrates that there will probably be many more mutations in this gene; their classification by functional relevance is the main task for an understanding of this gene's role in lipoprotein metabolism disorders.

These two genes also serve as good examples for the illustration of different methodological approaches to gene diagnostics. Defectes in the LDL-receptor gene are so diverse that, apart from populations with founder effects, individuals with receptor defects only rarely have a mutation in common. Consequently, a genetic diagnosis of FH is done indirectly by analysing the cosegregation of markers at this locus with the clinical phenotype. The absence of a cross-over event in five observed informative meioses results in an approximately 97% security of the diagnosis of FH. The problems with this type of diagnostic procedure are that it works only for phenotypes which are well separated from normal, and that it requires the analysis of a considerable number of family members. Consequently, less pronounced phenotypes escape from diagnosis with this method. To avoid misinterpretations carriers defined by LDL-cholesterol concentrations are above the 97th percentile of the sex- and age-matched population distribution curve while normals are required to have lower than 75th percentile concentrations. Persons with LDL-cholesterol between the 75th and 97th percentiles are excluded from analysis. Although currently available data do not allow us to speculate on the role of diagnostic sequencing in the diagnosis of FH, it is intriguing to speculate that eventually sequencing techniques might be fast enough for routine diagnostics, and that the association of a specific mutation with disease can be found by comparison with the content of a mutation database.

To show the presence or absence of a gene defect is much easier in FDB, where a single mutation is the only cause of the disease. Today's technology provides a number of methods suited for rapid, reliable, and economical detection of specific gene defects. Most of these procedures are based on the polymerase chain reaction (PCR)-mediated amplification of a specific part of the genome, which harbours the defect[11]. Subsequent analysis is done by hybridization of allele-specific aligonucleotides or by restriction fragment analysis. The use of allele-specific and mutagenic primers during PCR has helped to simplify gene diagnostics for routine procedures[12,13].

The above-mentioned mutations cause increased LDL-cholesterol levels. Mutations responsible for another CAD risk factor, low HDL-cholesterol, have also been identified. Defects resulting in the complete or near-complete absence of HDL-cholesterol from serum have been identified in the genes encoding for apolipoprotein A-I, an essential structural component of normal HDL, and lecithin: cholesterol acyl-transferase (LCAT), a plasma enzyme necessary for HDL matura-tion[14,15]. These defects are rare and consequently their diagnostic importance is low. They do, however, serve an important role for our understanding of how low HDL-cholesterol leads to increased CAD risk. The identification of apoA-I mutations as the structural basis for HDL deficiency has been reported in individuals with HDL deficiency as well as those without the disease. Familial HDL deficiency is usually not associated with CAD risk, when the underlying defect is located in the LCAT gene. It is not currently know if as yet unrecognized differences in the biochemical consequences of the mutations are responsible for this diversity in the associated clinical phenotypes, or if this is a consequence of the presence of the number and quality of additional risk factors. The absence of CAD from some HDL-deficient individuals has, however, shown that there is no direct and obligatory link between the biochemical marker and the clinical disease[16].

Since in hypercholesterolaemia the pathological agent is probably identified as LDL-cholesterol a reduction in plasma by any method is thought to be beneficial for the individual's health. In the case of HDL-cholesterol it is not currently understood whether there is a direct relationship to CAD or if it serves as a surrogate for an as yet unidentified pathological mechanism. Risk determination, as well as the development of therapeutic strategies, may thus rest much upon the identification of the underlying fault.

COMBINATIONS OF GENE DEFECTS

In addition to the above-mentioned lipoprotein metabolism disorders which are characterized by a clearly identifiable codominant segregation pattern, numerous gene defects with smaller phenotypic consequences have been identified. Some of these minor mutations have frequencies that are 10 times or more higher than those of the major mutations, assigning them an important role in overall phenotype variation. The ascertainment of the phenotypic effects of minor mutations cannot be done by vertical genetic analyses, since the deviations from normal mediated by these mutations are small, and because of frequent additional variations of the quantitative phenotype by external factors such as diet and lifestyle. In these cases horizontal analysis of the genetic influence is used. The necessity for a matched presence of often unknown factors with impact on the phenotype in question requires analysis of large numbers of cases.

Even though their use in individual medicine may be limited, an understanding of the role of frequent minor mutations is essential for our concept of the genetic architecture of cardiovascular diseases. Due to the high frequency of some minor mutations it can be expected that their interaction with each other, and with external factors, is responsible for a significant proportion of CAD risk. Examples for such minor effects include two frequent mutations in apoE (Cys112Arg and Arg158Cys) which affect serum LDL-cholesterol and HDL-cholesterol concentrations[17], a frequent mutation in CETP (IIe405Val)[18] and three mutations in lipoprotein lipase (Asp9Asn, Asn291Ser, Ser447End) which are all associated with changes in HDL-cholesterol and triglyceride concentrations[19–21]. Similar observations have been made for the allelic variation in apo(a)[22–24].

Apart from the possibility that a risk-associated intermediate phenotype is formed as the consequence of unfavourable interaction of these mutants with each other some of them (apoE:112Arg and apo(a):IEF-phenotypes) have been shown to aggravate the phenotypic consequences resulting from FH.

While in some cases with occurrence of myocardial infarction at young age monogenic lipoprotein metabolism disorders are observed, the majority of MI patients present with polygenic multifactorial disorders. In this context it is interesting to note that with increasing age there is a change in the contribution of different intermediate phenotypes to CAD formation (Fig. 1). This observation suggests that some mutations may be associated with early disease onset, while others are typically of the late-onset type.

SUMMARY AND PERSPECTIVES

The low incidence of myocardial infarctions observed after World War II has often been interpreted as resulting from profound differences in diet and lifestyle at that time. This concept has gained support from knowing that the expression of major risk factors for CAD development (namely diabetes mellitus, hypertension, and lipoprotein metabolism disorders), is also governed by the presence of external factors. As the genetic composition of humans has not since changed, it is evident that CAD is not purely the consequence of genetic anomalies but requires unfavourable interaction with environmental factors. it could thus be that the majority of negative genetic effects become visible in conjunction only with a disadvantageous lifestyle. The extent of debauchery an individual is allowed may thus largely be determined by one's gene map.

At present only a small fraction of risk-associated phenotypes can be explained by already known mutations. It can, however, be expected that more mutations in more genes will rapidly follow. Work aimed at the introduction of a system based on genetic variation for diagnosis and management of cardiovascular diseases is rapidly progressing.

References

1. Miller NE, Forde OH, Thelle DS, Mjos OD. The Tromso heart-study. High density lipoprotein and coronary heart-disease: a prospective case-control study. Lancet. 1977;965–68.
2. Castellu WP, Garrison RJ, Wilson PWF, Abbott TD, Kalousdian S, Kannel WB. Incidence of coronary heart disease and lipoprotein cholesterol levels. The Framingham Study. JAMA. 1986;256:2835–8.
3. Assmann G, Schulte H. Relation of high-density lipoprotein cholesterol and triglycerides to incidence of atherosclerotic coronary artery disease (the PROCAM experience). Am J Cardiol. 1992;70:733–7.
4. Sing CF, Moll PP. Genetics of atherosclerosis. Annu Rev Genet. 1990;24:171–87.
5. Brown MS, Goldstein JL. The hyperlipoproteinemias and other disorders of lipid metabolism. In: Isselbacher KJ, Adams RD, Braunwald E, Petersdorf RG, Wilson JD, editors. Harrison's principles of internal medicine, 12th ed. New York: McGraw-Hill; 1991.
6. Rust S, Funke H, Assmann G. Analysis of pooled samples from nearly 10000 individuals, with mutagenically separated PCR (MS-PCR) shows a significant overrepresentation of familial defective apoB-100 in coronary artery disease patients. Circulation, Suppl. 1992;86:420.
7. Hobbs HH, Brown MS, Goldstein JL. Molecular genetics of the LDL receptor gene in familial hypercholesterolemia. Hum Mutation. 1992;1:445–66.
8. Innerarity TL, Mahley RW, Weisgraber KH, et al. Familial defective apolipoprotein B-100; a mutation of apolipoprotein B that causes hypercholesterolemia. J Lipid Res. 1990;31:1337–49.
9. Pullinger CR, Hennessy LK, Chatterton JE, et al. Familial ligand-defective apolipoprotein B: identification of a new mutation that decreases LDL receptor binding affinity. J Clin Invest. 1995;95:1225–34.

10. Ludwig EH, Blackhart BD, Pierotti VR, et al. DNA sequence of the human apolipoprotein B gene. DNA. 1987;6:363–72.
11. Mullis K, Faloona F, Scharf S, Saiki R, Horn G, Erlich H. Specific enzymatic amplification of DNA in vitro: the polymerase chain reaction. Cold Spring Harbor Symp Quant Biol. 1986;51:263–73.
12. Newton CR, Graham A, Heptinstall LE, et al. Analysis of any point mutation in DNA. The amplification refractory system (ARMS). Nucl Acids Res. 1989;17:2503–16.
13. Rust S, Funke H, Assmann G. Mutagenically separated PCR (MS-PCR): a highly specific one step procedure for easy mutation detection. Nucl Acids Res. 1993;21:3623–9.
14. Assmann G, von Eckardstein A, Funke H. High density lipoproteins, reverse transport of cholesterol, and coronary artery disease. Insights from mutations. Circulation, Suppl. 1993;87:28–34.
15. Funke H, von Eckardstein A, Pritchard PH, et al. Genetic and phenotypic heterogeneity in familial lecithin: cholesterol acyltransferase (LCAT) deficiency. Six newly identified defective alleles further contribute to the structural hetero-geneity in this disease. J Clin Invest. 1993;91:677–83.
16. Römling R, von Eckardstein A, Funke H, et al. A nonsense mutation in the apolipoprotein A-I gene is associated with high density lipoprotein deficiency and periorbital xanthelasmas. Arterioscler Thromb. 1994;14:1915–22.
17. Dallongeville J, Lussier-Cacan S, Davignon J. Modulation of plasma triglyceride levels by apoE phenotype: a meta-analysis. J Lipid Res. 1992;33:447–54.
18. Funke H, Wiebusch W, Fuer L, et al. Identification of mutations in the cholesterol ester transfer protein in Europeans with elevated high density lipoprotein cholesterol. Circulation. 1994;90:I-241.
19. Reymer PWA, Gagné E, Groenemeyer BE, et al. A lipoprotein lipase mutation (Asn291Ser) is associated with reduced HDL cholesterol levels in premature atherosclerosis. Nature Genet. 1995;10 (In press).
20. Funke H, Assmann G. The lowdown on lipoprotein lipase. Nature Genet. 1995;10 (In press).
21. Mailly F, Tugrul Y, Reymer PWA, et al. A common variant in the gene for lipoprotein lipase (Asp9→Asn): functional implications and prevalence in normal and hyperlipidemic subjects. Arterioscler Thromb Vascul Biol. 1995;15:468–78.
22. Lackner C, Boerwinkle E, Leffert CC, Rahmig T, Hobbs HH. Molecular basis of apolipoprotein (a) isoform size heterogeneity as revealed by pulsed-field gel electrophoresis. J Clin Invest. 1991;87:2153–61.
23. Cohen JC, Chiesa G, Hobbs HH. Sequence polymorphism in the apolipoprotei-n(a) gene. Evidence for dissociation between apolipoprotein(a) size and plasma lipoprotein(a) levels. J Clin Invest. 1993;91:1630–6.
24. Sandholzer C, Saha N, Kark JD, et al. Apo(a) isoforms predict risk for coronary heart disease. A study in six populations. Arterioscler Thromb. 1992;12:1214–26.

2

Role of high density lipoprotein subclasses in reverse cholesterol transport

A. VON ECKARDSTEIN, Y. HUANG and G. ASSMANN

INTRODUCTION

Several epidemiological and clinical studies have demonstrated the inverse correlation between the plasma concentration of high density lipoprotein (HDL) cholesterol and the risk of myocardial infarction (reviewed in ref. 1). The ability of HDL to protect the vessel wall from atherosclerosis has usually been explained by the reverse cholesterol transport model (reviewed in ref. 2) in which HDL mediates the flux of excess cholesterol from peripheral cells to the liver. HDL-cholesterol levels are determined by environmental and genetic factors. The influence of genes on the variation of HDL-cholesterol levels has been estimated to account for up to 50%, but only rare defects in the genes of apolipoprotein (apo)A-I and lecithin:cholesterol acyltransferase (LCAT) could be made responsible for familially low HDL-cholesterol levels[3]. Despite the virtual absence of HDL, several homozygotes for apoA-I deficiency, LCAT deficiency, and fish-eye disease, but also patients with Tangier disease or unclassified forms of HDL deficiency did not present with premature atherosclerosis[3–6]. Family histories of these patients did not indicate any increased prevalence of coronary heart disease (CHD) events, although heterozygotes for various defects in the genes of apoA-I and LCAT, as well as obligate heterozygotes for Tangier disease, usually have HDL-cholesterol levels below the 10th percentile of sex- and age-matched controls[3,5,6]. These clinical observations have questioned a direct anti-atherogenic role of HDL. HDL, however, include structurally and functionally heterogeneous lipoproteins which can be differentiated on the basis of density, size, charge and apolipoprotein composition[7]. During recent years, experiments of our and other investigators' laboratories have yielded a large body of evidence show-

17

ing that minor subfractions of HDL which escape the quantification of HDL-cholesterol are important contributors to reverse cholesterol transport.

ELECTROPHORETIC DIFFERENTIATION OF HDL SUBCLASSES

Agarose gel electrophoresis differentiates a quantitatively minor proportion of HDL with preβ- (i.e. α_2-)mobility from the bulk of HDL which migrates with the α_1-globulins[8,9]. Both fractions contain apoA-I. The different electrophoretic mobility of these particles is essentially caused by differences in the content of cholesterol and phosphatidylinositol[10]. Non-denaturing polyacrylamide gradient gel electrophoresis (PAGGE) of particles which have been pre-separated by agarose gel electrophoresis and subsequent anti-apoA-I-immunoblotting differentiates by size preβ_1-LpA-I, preβ_2-LpA-I, and preβ_3-LpA-I as well as α-LpA-I$_3$ (Stokes diameter 7.2–8.8 nm) and α-LpA-I$_2$ (Stokes diameter 8.8–12 nm)[11–13]. Anti-apoE-immunoblotting of two-dimensional PAGGE gels identifies the majority of HDL-associated apoE in a particle with electrophoretic α-mobility. A minor proportion of apoE migrates in a particle with electrophoretic γ-mobility which is termed γ-LpE[14].

ROLE OF HDL SUBCLASSES

Pulse-chase incubations of plasma with [^{3}H]cholesterol-laden fibroblasts and subsequent two-dimensional PAGGE identified both preβ_1-LpA-I and γ-LpE as initial acceptors of cell-derived cholesterol (see below)[10,11,14]. ApoA-I and apoE, respectively, constitute the only proteins. In normal plasma the amount of [^{3}H]cholesterol accumulating in γ-LpE equals or even exceeds the amount in preβ_1-LpA-I[14,15]. Plasma which has been depleted from apoA-I by anti-apoA-I-immunoaffinity chromatography[16], as well as plasmas from apoA-I-deficient patients, are reduced by approximately 50% in their ability to take up cell-derived [^{3}H]cholesterol[15]. This suggests that apoA-I-free lipoproteins, especially γ-LpE, considerably contribute to the uptake of cellular cholesterol into plasma. The importance of γ-LpE for the uptake of cell-derived cholesterol into plasma is also highlighted by the effects of the apoE polymorphism on both the formation of γ-LpE and cholesterol efflux.

18

We previously found that γ-LpE is present only in plasmas of individuals who carry at least one apoE3 allele[16]. Plasmas containing apoE3 released [^{3}H]cholesterol from fibroblasts into both γ-LpE and preβ_1-LpA-I. Plasmas from homozygotes for apoE2 or apoE4 took up cell-derived [^{3}H]cholesterol only into preβ_1-LpA-I. Compared to apoE3-containing plasmas, samples of homozygotes for apoE2 or apoE4 were reduced by 35–40% in their ability to release cholesterol from cells. This again demonstrates that γ-LpE is responsible for the majority of the residual activity of apoA-I-deficient plasma to release cholesterol from cells. Moreover, these data suggest that genetic variation in apoE affects cholesterol efflux from cells[16]. However, heterogeneity may exist with respect to the subcellular compartments of cholesterol which are depleted by the various HDL subfractions. Thus, the preβ_1-LpA-I-dependent efflux of [^{3}H]cholesterol is sensitive towards protease pre-treatment of cells. Therefore, Kawano and colleagues hypothesized that this part of cholesterol efflux depends on the interaction of preβ_1-LpA-I with a cell-surface protein[17]. In the future it will be important to compare preβ_1-LpA-I and γ-LpE regarding their ability to release cholesterol from distinct subcellular pools.

To date the transfer and esterification of cell-derived cholesterol in plasma has been analysed by experiments which considered only the involvement of apoA-I containing lipoproteins. In these experiments cellular cholesterol taken up by preβ_1-LpA-I appeared to be transferred to LDL via preβ_2-LpA-I → preβ_3-LpA-I → α-LpA-I[12]. Some cholesterol is esterified in preβ_3-LpA-I which contains CETP, LCAT and apoD[18]. The majority of cholesterol is esterified in α-LpA-I after re-transfer from LDL[12,19]. To date it is not known by which route cholesterol is transferred from γ-LpE to LDL. Neither is it known how cholesterol is transferred between the various HDL subclasses. Incubation of plasma leads to the disappearance of preβ_1-LpA-I[20]. This suggests that preβ_1-LpA-I is converted into other particles. Conversion of preβ_1-LpA-I would provide a flux of cholesterol. The mechanism and the product of preβ_1-LpA-I conversion are as yet unknown. LCAT appears to be involved but cannot fully explain the conversion[21].

GENERATION AND CONVERSION OF HDL SUBCLASSES

By contrast, several mechanisms have been described which investigated the generation of preβ_1-LpA-I. HDL with preβ-mobility predominate in cell culture media of hepatocytes as well as in the lymph[22,23]. Incubation of lipid-free apoA-I with various cells generates a particle with electrophoretic preβ-mobility[21,24]. Preβ-LpA-I is also generated by the incubation of HDL_2 with CETP or hepatic lipase[25,26]. Incubation of HDL_3 with phospholipid transfer protein (PLTP) produces HDL_2 and a smaller particle which we recently identified as preβ$_1$-LpA-I[27–29]. Thus, conversion of preβ$_1$-LpA-I into mature HDL introduces preβ$_1$-LpA-I and cell-derived cholesterol into a cycle in which cholesterol is esterified and targeted to the liver, and in which preβ$_1$-LpA-I particles are newly generated.

γ-LpE are found in cell culture media of hepatocytes and macrophages[14] and can be generated by the incubation of lipid-free apoE with fibroblasts. Thereby, γ-LpE also resembles nascent HDL. Its metabolic fate is not known.

REVERSE CHOLESTEROL TRANSPORT IN FAMILIAL HDL DEFICIENCY

In plasma from patients with apoA-I deficiency, Tangier disease (TD), familial LCAT-deficiency, and fish eye disease (FED), the distribution of LpA-I subfractions differs considerably from that in normal plasma[15]: LpA-I are absent in apoA-I deficiency. In plasmas from patients with TD, FED and LCAT deficiency, preβ$_1$-LpA-I and preβ$_2$-LpA-I, but not preβ$_3$-LpA-I, are present; α-LpA-I is undetectable in TD plasma. Some small α-LpA-I, i.e. α-LpA-I$_3$, are detectable in plasmas from patients with FED or LCAT deficiency. All plasmas contain γ-LpE[5]. In apoA-I deficiency only γ-LpE takes up cell-derived [³H]cholesterol. This is accompanied by a 50% decrease in the plasma uptake of cellular [³H]UC during a 1-minute pulse. In TD, familial LCAT deficiency, and FED, cell-derived [³H]UC was taken up by both preβ$_1$-LpA-I and γ-LpE. Compared to normal plasma the uptake of cellular [³H]UC after a 1 minute pulse in plasmas from these patients was reduced by 28% (FED), 36% (TD) and 21% (LCAT deficiency)[15].

In normal plasma, cell-derived cholesterol is esterified either in preβ$_3$-LpA-I which contains CETP, LCAT and apoD[12,18], or in α-LpA-I after re-transfer from LDL[12,19]. In HDL-deficient plasmas cell-derived [³H]cholesterol is more rapidly transferred to LDL than in normal plasma. LCAT-deficienct plasma does not esterify cell-derived [³H]cholesterol. In FED plasma, esterification of [³H]UC takes place in LDL. In plasma from patients with apoA-I deficiency and TD, however, ester-ification occurs in lipoproteins free of apoA-I and apoB; the transfer of [^{3}H]cholesteryl esters to LDL is enhanced compared to normal plasma[15].

Net cholesterol efflux from fibroblasts into plasma is decreased to 52%, 88%, 66% and 40% for apoA-I deficiency, TD, FED and LCAT deficiency, respectively, as compared to normoalphalipoproteinaemic plasma. Removal of LpB from plasma of patients with apoA-I deficiency, TD, LCAT deficiency, and FED further decreases net cholesterol efflux rates to 23%, 16%, 28% and 36%, respectively, compared to 61% in normoalphalipoproteinaemic control plasma.

CONCLUSION

Our findings indicate that minor HDL subfractions such as preβ$_1$-LpA-I and γ-LpE, which are present even in HDL-deficient plasmas, are functionally important. Moreover, the failure of apoE4 to form γ-LpE may be pathogenetically involved in the increased cardiovascular risk of individuals with apoE4.

Acknowledgements

The work of Dr Arnold von Eckardstein is supported by grants from Wissenschaftsminsterium Nordrhein-Westfalen (Bennigsen-Foerder-Preis) and Deutsche Forschungsgemeinschaft (Ec116,3-1).

References

1. Gordon D, Rifkind BM. Current concepts: high density lipoproteins – the clinical implications of recent studies. N Engl J Med. 1989;321:1311–15.
2. Tall AR. Plasma high density lipoproteins. Metabolism and relationship to atherogenesis. J Clin Invest. 1990;86:379–84.
3. Assmann G, von Eckardstein A, Funke H. High density lipoproteins, reverse transport of cholesterol and coronary heart disease: insights from mutants. Circulation. 1993;87(Suppl.III):28–34.
4. Serfaty-Lacrosniere C, Civeira F, Lanzberg A, et al. Homozygous Tangier disease and cardiovascular disease. Atherosclerosis. 1994;107:85–98.
5. Assmann G, von Eckardstein A, Brewer HB Jr. Familial high density lipoprotein deficiency: Tangier disease. In: Scriver CR, Beaudet AL, Sly WS, Valle D, editors.

The metabolic basis of inherited disease. New York: McGraw-Hill Information Services, 7th edn; 1995:2053–72.

6. Norum KR, Assmann G, Glomset JA. Familial lecithin:cholesterol acyltransferase deficiency and fish-eye disease. In: Scriver CR, Beaudet AL, Sly WS, Valle D, editors. The metabolic basis of inherited disease. New York: McGraw-Hill Information Services, 7th edn; 1995:1933–51.
7. von Eckardstein A, Huang Y, Assmann G. Physiological role and clinical relevance of high density lipoprotein subclasses. Curr Opin Lipidol. 1994;5:404–16.
8. Fielding CJ, Fielding PE. A cholesteryl ester transfer complex in human plasma. Proc Natl Acad Sci USA. 1980;77:3327–31.
9. Kunitake ST, La Sala KI, Kane JP. Apolipoprotein A-I containing lipoproteins with prebeta electrophoretic mobility. J Lipid Res. 1985;26: 549–55.
10. Davidson WS, Sparks DL, Lund-Katz S, Philips MC. The molecular basis for the difference of charge between preβ- and α-migrating high density lipoproteins. J Biol Chem. 1994;269:8959–65.
11. Castro GR, Fielding CJ. Early incorporation of cell-derived cholesterol into pre-β-migrating high density lipoprotein. Biochemistry. 1988;27:25–9.
12. Huang Y, von Eckardstein A, Assmann G. Cell-derived cholesterol cycles between different HDLs and LDL for its effective esterification in plasma. Arterioscler Thromb. 1993;13:445–58.
13. Asztalos BF, Sloop CH, Wong L, Roheim PS. Two-dimensional electrophoresis of plasma lipoproteins: recognition of new apoA-I containing subpopulations. Biochim Biophys Acta. 1993;1169:291–300.
14. Huang Y, von Eckardstein A, Wu S, Maeda N, Assmann G. A plasma lipoprotein containing only apolipoprotein E and with γ-mobility on electrophoresis releases cholesterol from cells. Proc Natl Acad Sci USA. 1994;91:1834–8.
15. von Eckardstein AY, Huang Y, Wu S, Funke H, Noseda G, Assmann G. Uptake, transfer, and esterification of cell-derived cholesterol in plasma of patients with different forms of familial high density lipoprotein deficiency. Arterioscler Thromb Vasc Biol. 1994;15:691–703.
16. Huang Y, von Eckardstein A, Wu S, Assmann G. Effects of the apolipoprotein E-polymorphism on uptake and transfer of cell-derived cholesterol in plasma. Submitted 1994.
17. Kawano M, Miida T, Fielding CJ, Fielding PE. Quantitation of preβ-HDL-dependent and nonspecific components of the total efflux of cellular cholesterol and phospholipid. Biochemistry. 1993;32:5025–8.
18. Francone OL, Gurakar A, Fielding CJ. Distribution and functions of lecithin:cholesterol acyltransferase and cholesterol ester transfer protein in plasma lipoproteins. J Biol Chem. 1989;264:7066–72.
19. Miida T, Fielding CJ, Fielding PE. Mechanism of transfer of LDL-derived free cholesterol to HDL subfractions in human plasma. Biochemistry. 1990;29:10469–74.
20. Miida T, Kawano M, Fielding CJ, Fielding PE. Regulation of the concentration of pre-β high density lipoprotein in normal plasma by cell membranes and lecithin:cholesterol acyltransferase activity. Biochemistry. 1992;31:11112–17.
21. Huang Y, von Eckardstein A, Wu S, Assmann G. Generation of preβ1-high density lipoprotein (HDL) and conversin into α-HDL: evidence for disturbed preβ1-HDL conversion in Tangier disease. Submitted 1994.
22. Lefevre M, Sloop CH, Roheim PS. Characterization of dog prenodal peripheral lymph lipoproteins. Evidence for the peripheral formation of lipoprotein-unasso-

22

ciated apoA-I with slow preβ-electrophoretic mobility. J Lipid Res. 1988;29:1139–48.

23. Forte TM, Goth-Goldstein R, Nordhausen RW, McCall MR. Apolipoprotein A-I-cell membrane interaction: extracellular assembly of heterogeneous nascent HDL particles. J Lipid Res. 1993;34:317–24.

24. Hara H, Yokoyama S. Role of apolipoproteins in cholesterol efflux from macrophages to lipid microemulsion: proposal of a putative model for the pre-β-high density lipoprotein pathway. Biochemistry. 1992;31:2040–6.

25. Barrans A, Collet X, Barbaras R, et al. Hepatic lipase induces the formation of preβ₁-high density lipoprotein (HDLO) from triacylglycerol-rich HDL_2. J Biol Chem. 1994;269:11572–7.

26. Hennessy LK, Kunitake ST, Kane JP. Apolipoprotein A-I-containing lipoproteins, with or without apolipoprotein A-II, as progenitors of preβ-high density lipoprotein particles. Biochemistry. 1993;32:5759–65.

27. Jauhiainen M, Metso J, Pahlman R, Blomqvist S, van Tol A, Ehnholm C. Human plasma phospholipid transfer protein causes high density lipoprotein conversion. J Biol Chem. 1993;268:4032–6.

28. Tu AY, Nishida HI, Nishida T. High density lipoprotein conversion mediated by human phospholipid transfer protein. J Biol Chem. 1993;268:23098–105.

29. Von Eckardstein A, Jauhiainen M, Huang Y, et al. Conversion of high density lipoproteins (HDL) by phospholipid transfer protein generates prebeta₁-HDL. Submitted 1994.

3

Connection between cholesterol efflux and atherosclerosis

J.C. FRUCHART, C. DE GETEIRE, B. DELFY and G.R. CASTRO

Epidemiological studies have consistently demonstrated that the plasma high density lipoproteins (HDL) are inversely correlated with the risk of coronary artery disease (CAD)[1,2]. HDL are highly heterogeneous with respect to the hydrated density, size and composition of the particles. The major apolipoprotein (apo) in HDL, apoA-I, has been shown to have a strong inverse correlation with risk of CAD[3-5], whereas an inverse correlation with apoA-II levels has not been consistently demonstrated[3]. It has been shown by several laboratories that there are several subclasses of apoA-I containing particles. The two major subclasses include particles that contain both apoA-I and apoA-II (termed LpA-I, A-II) and those that contain apoA-I but not apoA-II (termed LpA-I). Apo-specific particles can be isolated by use of immunoaffinity columns with anti-apoA-I or anti-apoA-II antibody[6,7].

A number of studies indicate that LpA-I and LpA-I:A-II are metabolically distinct and may perform different functions. ApoA-I injected as part of LpA-I particles is catabolized at a higher rate than apoA-I injected as part of LpA-I:A-II particles[8].

Of considerable significance was the finding that two proteins stimulating reverse cholesterol transport lecithin:cholesterol acyltransferase (LCAT) and cholesteryl ester transfer protein (CETP) are mainly present in LpA-I particles[9].

The purpose of this chapter is to review the role of these different apoA-I containing particles in reverse cholesterol transport, and to demonstrate a connection between cholesterol efflux and atherosclerosis risk.

It has been reported[10,11] that human plasma LpA-I is a potent agonist for the promotion of cholesterol mass efflux from cholesterol-loaded

25

Ob1771 cells, a mouse adipocyte cell line. However, human plasma LpA-I:A-II particles were unable to reduce the cell cholesterol content and, in fact, blocked the ability of LpA-I in promoting cholesterol efflux. Since both particles appear to compete for the same high-affinity binding sites on the cell surface, it was suggested that LpA-I:A-II particles are antagonists and LpA-I particles are agonists for cholesterol efflux from the Ob1771 cell line[11]. In contrast, other studies using different cell types have shown that LpA-I and LpA-I:A-II are equally effective in promoting efflux of plasma membrane or lysosomal cholesterol[12-14]; these conflicting reports suggest that the interaction of LpA-I:A-II particles with cells, and its effect on cholesterol efflux, differ between cell types and may be influenced by several factors that modulate transport of cellular cholesterol.

To investigate whether the apolipoprotein composition is important for the delivery of cholesterol esters to the liver, and for the kinetics of bile acid formation, the fate of cholesterol esters of LpA-I and LpA-I:A-II were compared in the rat[15]. The data indicated that, even when both particles were able to selectively deliver cholesterol esters to the liver, the cholesterol esters delivered by LpA-I were more efficiently coupled to the bile acid synthesis.

The results in transgenic mice with primarily human LpA-I particles confirmed the protective role of apoA-I for atherosclerosis while the overexpression of human apoA-II in human apoA-I transgenic mice appears to promote rather than retard aortic fatty streak development[16]. In order to examine the biochemical mechanisms underlying these *in-vivo* observations we have tested sera from human A-I transgenic and human apoA-I/apoA-II transgenic mice for participation in cholesterol efflux *in vitro*. Analysis of cholesterol efflux from Fu5AH cells according to the method described by Moya et al.[17] revealed that the serum from human A-I transgenic mice produces a significantly higher level of cholesterol efflux than the human apoA-I/apoA-II transgenic mice (data unpublished). This study shows for the first time a correlation between *in-vivo* atherogenesis and *in-vitro* cholesterol efflux. Two other studies demonstrate that apoA-I, the most abundant protein in HDL, plays a crucial role in the mechanism of reverse cholesterol transport. Using natural variants of apoA-I[18] and an immunochemical approach with mapped anti-apoA-I monoclonal antibodies[19], we have shown that the region of apoA-I around amino acid 165 is involved in their interaction with cells. The use of a synthetic tetrameric peptide that mimics properties of apoA-I allowed us to confirm the importance of this particular region in the biological role of apoA-I[20].

References

1. Miller GJ, Miller NE. Plasma high density lipoprotein concentration and development of ischaemic heart disease. Lancet. 1975;1:16.
2. Gordon DJ, Rifkind BM. High density lipoprotein: the clinical implications of recent studies. N Engl J Med. 1989;321:1311.
3. Miller NE. Associations of high density lipoprotein subclasses and apolipoproteins with ischemic heart disease and coronary atherosclerosis. Am Heart J. 1987;113:589.
4. Brunzell JD, Sniderman AD, Albers JJ, Kwiterowich PO. Apoproteins B and A-I and coronary heart disease in humans. Atherosclerosis. 1984;4:79.
5. Maciejko JJ, Holmes DR, Kottke BA, Zinsmeister AR, Dinh DM, Mao SJ. Apolipoprotein A-I as a marker for angiographically assessed coronary artery disease. N Engl J Med. 1983;309:385.
6. Cheung MC, Albers JJ. Characterization of lipoprotein particles isolated by immunoaffinity chromatography. Particles containing A-I and A-II and particles containing A-I but no A-II. J Biol Chem. 1984;259:12201.
7. James RW, Hochstrasser D, Tissot JD, et al. Protein heterogeneity of lipoprotein particles containing apolipoprotein A-I without apolipoprotein A-II and apolipoprotein A-I with apolipoprotein A-II isolated from human plasma. J Lipid Res. 1988;29:1557.
8. Rader DY, Castro GR, Zech LA, Fruchart JC, Brewer HB Jr. In vivo metabolism of apolipoprotein A-I on high density lipoprotein particles LpA-I and LpA-I:A-II. J Lipid Res. 1991;32:1849.
9. Cheung MC, Wolf AC, Lum KD, Tollefson JH, Albers JJ. Distribution and localization of lecithin cholesterol acyltransferase and cholesterol ester transfer activity in A-I containing lipoproteins. J Lipid Res. 1986;27:1135.
10. Barbaras R, Puchois P, Fruchart JC, Ailhaud G. Cholesterol efflux from cultured adipose cells is mediated by LpA-I particles but not by LpA-I:A-II particles. Biochem Biophys Res Commun. 1987;142:63.
11. Barkia AR, Barbaras R, Ghalim N, Puchois P, Ailhaud G, Fruchart JC. Effect of different apo A-I containing lipoprotein particles on reverse cholesterol transport in fat cells. Horm Metab Res. 1988;Suppl.19:10.
12. Johnson WY, Kilsdonk EPC, Van Tol A, Phillips MC, Rothblat GH. Cholesterol efflux from cells to immunopurified subfractions of human high density lipoprotein:LpA-I and LpA-I:A-II. J Lipid Res. 1991;32:1993.
13. Ohta T, Nakamura R, Ikeda Y, et al. Differential effect of subspecies of lipoprotein containing apolipoprotein A-I on cholesterol efflux from cholesterol loaded macrophages: functional correlation with lecithin cholesterol acyltransferase. Biochim Biophys Acta. 1992;1165:119.
14. Oikawa S, Mendez A, Oram JF, Bierman EL, Cheung MC. Effects of high density lipoprotein particles containing apo A-I with or without apo A-II on intracellular cholesterol efflux. Biochim Biophys Acta. 1993;1165:327.
15. Pieters MN, Castro GR, Schouten D, et al. Cholesterol esters selectively delivered in vivo by high density lipoprotein subclass LpA-I to rat liver are processed faster

into bile acids than are LpA-I:A-II delivered cholesterol esters. Biochem J. 1993;292:819.

16. Schultz JR, Verstugft JG, Goug EL, Nichols AV, Rubin EM. Protein composition determines the anti-atherogenic properties of high density lipoproteins in transgenic mice. Nature. 1993;365:761.

17. de la Llera Moya M, Atger V, Paul JL, et al. A cell culture system for screening human serum for ability to promote cellular cholesterol efflux; relationship between serum components and efflux, esterification and transfer. Arteriosclerosis Thromb. 1994;14:1056.

18. Von Eckardstein A, Castro GR, Wybranska J, et al. Interaction of reconstituted high density lipoprotein discs containing human apolipoprotein A-I (apo A-I) variants with murine adipocytes and macrophages: evidence for reduced cholesterol efflux promotion by apo A-I (Pro[165] Arg). J Biol Chem. 1993;268:2616.

19. Luchoomun J, Theret N, Clavey V, et al. Structural domain of apolipoprotein A-I involved in its interaction with cells. Biochim Biophys Acta. 1994;1212:319.

20. Luchoomun J, Demoor L, Tartar A, et al. A synthetic tetrameric peptide that mimics properties of apo A-I. Circulation. 1993(Suppl.88):abstr. 2482.

4

HDLC as a therapeutic target in coronary disease: current concepts and future directions

B.G. BROWN, XUE-QIAO ZHAO, V.M.G. MAHER, A. CHAIT, M. CHEUNG, L.D. FISHER and J. ALBERS

INTRODUCTION

Gordon et al.[1] in 1977, first drew our attention to the idea that, within the spectrum of cholesterol-containing particles, HDL-cholesterol (HDLC) was associated with reduced risk of coronary heart disease. Since then, HDL have received a great amount of attention. There is now emerging evidence to support the concepts that HDL-related measures are as important as LDL-related ones in predicting vascular events. Furthermore, pharmacological or genetic modification of certain plasma HDL subfractions appears to hold promise for clinical benefits that are comparable to, or perhaps exceed, those of LDLC reduction.

HDLC AS A RISK FACTOR FOR CLINICAL CORONARY EVENTS

A recent insightful analysis by Gordon et al.[2] puts the importance of HDLC as a cardiovascular (CV) risk factor in a clear perspective. The independent contribution to CV and CHD risk was assessed by comparable statistical methods, using data from the Framingham Heart Study (FHS)[3], the Lipid Research Clinics Prevalence Follow-Up Study (LRCPF)[4], and from control group patients in the LRC Coronary Primary Prevention Trial (CPPT)[5] and the Multiple Risk Factor Intervention Trial (MRFIT)[6]. For unselected subjects in these studies,

HDLC averaged 45 mg/dl among men and 57 mg/dl among women. Coronary heart disease (CHD) incidence was defined as the annual rate of occurrence of fatal and non-fatal myocardial infarction, sudden cardiac death, and acute coronary insufficiency. The total sample from these four studies in this analysis was about 24 000 patients. For each of these studies, vital statistics at the time of the follow-up analysis were available in 97%, 99.6%, 100% and 99.7% of the cohorts, respectively. In all cases, manganese heparin precipitation was used in measuring HDLC.

The composite epidemiological evidence for HDLC-associated risk, after adjusting for other risk covariates including smoking, systolic blood pressure, age, body mass index, and LDLC, by proportional hazards regression, may be summarized as follows:

A 1.0 mg/dl increment in HDLC was associated with a significant CHD risk decrement of 2% in men (FHS, CPPT, MRFIT) and 3% in women (FHS). In LRCPF, where only fatal outcomes were documented, a 1.0 mg/dl increment in HDLC was associated with a significant 3.7% (men) and 4.7% (women) decrement in cardio-vascular disease mortality rates.

The 95% confidence intervals for these decrements in CHD and CVD mortality all contain the range 1.9–2.9%. This inverse relationship of CHD risk to HDLC is continuous; is independent of the concentration of VLDL and/or LDL; is independent of non-lipid risk factors for CHD such as cigarette smoking, blood pressure, glucose intolerance and obesity; applies to CHD mortality as well as morbidity; is present in both middle-aged and elderly subjects; applies to both sexes; and applies to subjects with, as well as those without, a previous history of myocardial ischaemia. HDLC levels were essentially unrelated to non-cardiovascular disease mortality[2].

These data may be used to predict ($e^{-c\Delta HDL}$) that a pharmacologically achievable 10 mg/dl increase in HDLC would translate to a 19% (men) and 26% (women) reduction in overall coronary disease incidence and to 31% and 38% reductions, respectively, in cardiovascular mortality risk. The independent effect of LDL reduction on CAD risk (1.5% risk reduction for 1% LDL reduction)[5], is of comparable magnitude.

In another large population-based study[7], the relative risk of MI in 246 case-matched male physicians was strongly and independently predicted by HDLC and total cholesterol (TC). Other sub-fractions did not add to the predictive value of the TC/HDLC ratio. After adjusting for age, smoking, obesity and diabetes, a one unit change in this ratio resulted in a 53% mean reduction in MI risk. Importantly, higher HDLC was more beneficial among those with lower TC.

The relation of HDL subclass to severity and rate of progression of coronary atherosclerosis was investigated in 60 men who had survived MI before age 45 and had then undergone two arteriograms separated by 4–7 years. Five HDL subclasses were separated by gradient gel electrophoresis and major lipoprotein classes separated by preparative ultracentrifugation. The largest HDL particles, the HDL2b subclass, had significant inverse correlations with disease severity and disease progression. On further evaluation, this relationship was exceptionally strong and exclusive to patients with normal VLDL triglyceride levels. There was no such association between HDL2b and CAD in those with hypertriglyceridaemia[8]. These retrospective studies require further confirmation.

HDLC AS A DETERMINANT OF ATHEROSCLEROSIS PROGRESSION

Several studies have addressed the role of HDLC in the angiographic progression of coronary disease[9,10]. In the Cholesterol-Lowering Atherosclerosis Study (CLAS) the apo CIII content of HDL, relative to that in VLDL, was a protective factor in the diet-treated control group[9]. Phillips et al.[10] report that HDLC is inversely, and IDL + VLDL remnants are positively, associated with quantitative measures of atherosclerosis progression. In the FATS trial[11], the change in HDLC from baseline levels to mean values in treatment was strongly correlated with disease change. This multivariate analysis of all potential risk factors for disease progression in FATS identified four independent and significant contributors to prediction of change in proximal disease severity:

$$\Delta\%S \text{ prox} = +0.035 \ (\%\Delta LDLC) -0.045 \ (\%\Delta HDLC) +0.15 \ (\%\Delta BPs) \\ -0.8 \ (\Delta ST_{ETT}) + 1.2 \\ r = 0.47, \ p < 0.001$$

where $\Delta\%S$ prox is mean change in measured proximal disease (percentage stenosis) severity over the 2.5 year treatment period, $(\%\Delta\ldots$ is percentage change in either LDLC, HDLC or systolic blood

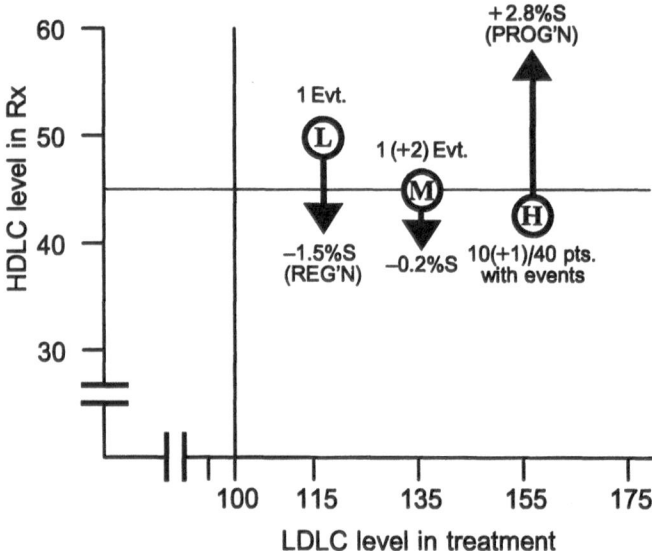

Fig. 1. Relationships among LDLC, HDLC, progression, regression and clinical cardiovascular events in FATS. Events are classified in terms of their frequency among 120 patients who completed the follow-up arteriogram and (in parenthesis) among those who died (1 patient) or quit the study early ($n = 25$). Patients are subclassified in terms of 3 terciles of predicted proximal disease change according to the formula in the text (L = low risk; M = mid-risk; H = high risk). Benefits to arteries and events are significantly associated with both reduced LDLC and increased HDLC.

pressure, and ST_{ETT} is the ST segment change (depression is negative) on baseline treadmill testing. Of note the magnitude of the LDLC and HDLC coefficients are comparable, with opposite sign; this, in effect, says that a 20% increase in HDLC is as beneficial (or more so) to proximal disease as a 20% reduction in LDLC. Figure 1 shows the interrelationship between in-treatment LDLC and HDLC levels, measured coronary stenosis progression (or regression) and clinical cardiovascular events for terciles of the above predictive function among 120 patients who completed FATS (or among 146 enrolled). Finally, a subgroup analysis in FATS[12] shows that patients with LDLC in the 130–160 mg/dl range, commonly with elevated triglycerides and low HDL, are at greatest risk of atherosclerosis progression and clinical events, and most likely to benefit from intensive therapy.

32

Table 1 Familial HDL deficiency states. Not all conditions with low HDLC are associated with increased coronary artery disease (CAD) risk.

	Heterozygotes HDLC[a] ApoA-I[b]		Homozygotes HDLC ApoA-I		CAD risk
ApoA-I/C-III deficiency	27	76	2	0	+++
Isolated hypoalphalipo-proteinaemia	26	70	0	0	+++
Tangier disease	27	55	2	1	0 (+)
Classic LCAT deficiency	32	112	4	33	0
Fish eye disease	33	120	7	38	0
ApoA-I_Milano	11	13	(none yet found)		0

[a]Median HDLC in the normal population is 45 mg/dl for men and 55 mg/dl for women

[b]Median apoA-I in the normal population is 130 mg/dl for men and 145 mg/dl for women

EVIDENCE FROM GENETIC HDLC DEFICIENCY DISORDERS

In humans with familial deficiency of HDLC and normal triglycerides, apoA-I synthesis is reduced and CAD risk is increased[12]. More rarely, major gene deletions at the apoA-I–A-IV–C-III locus are associated with severe premature CAD[14]. Other, but not all, genetic disorders with low apoA-I and HDLC are associated with premature CAD, suggesting a definite, but complex, relationship[15,16] (see Table 1).

Ath-2, a gene determining atherosclerosis susceptibility and HDL levels, has been identified in mice[17]. Furthermore, transgenic mice over-expressing human apoA-I show elevated plasma HDLC[18,19]. Conversely, transgenic mice over-expressing mouse apoA-II had elevated HDLC but nevertheless, exhibited increased atherosclerotic lesion development as compared to non-transgenic mice on comparable low-fat chow diets. Male, but not female, transgenic mice had increased aortic lesions when maintained on an atherogenic high-fat diet[20]. Based on these studies, we examined the effects of these two apoproteins on change in angiographically quantified CAD in the FATS patients[21]. To summarize, apoA-I levels during treatment correlated inversely with %S ($r = 0.26$, $p = 0.005$). Conversely, apoA-II levels correlated positively ($r = 0.21$, $p = 0.092$). The ratio, apoA-I/A-II was the best predictor of

$\Delta\%S$ ($r = -0.42$, $p < 0.0001$). Disease change correlated with HDL2 levels during treatment, but not with HDL3. These data confirm the anti-atherogenicity of apoA-I and show for the first time that apoA-II is pro-atherogenic in humans.

CAD RISK AMONG HDLC SIZE SUBPOPULATIONS

Cheung and co-workers[22] have pioneered an immunoaffinity column method for separation of HDL particles containing apoA-I, but no apo-A-II, from those containing both apoA-I and apoA-II. Non-denaturing gradient gel electrophoresis then provides a particle size profile of each subgroup. Based on the clustering of particle sizes from normolipidae-mic subjects, four intervals (7.0–8.2 nm, 8.2–9.2 nm, 9.2–11.2 nm and 11.2–17.0 nm) were devised to describe the particle size profile of each subgroup and to facilitate comparison among individuals. These techni-ques have permitted the examination of HDL beyond its total lipid and protein content to determine whether certain physical characteristics contribute independently to the prediction of CAD risk, or are altered in a consistent manner by lipid-lowering therapy.

Cheung et al.[23] examined the size profiles of HDL particles in nine normolipidaemic (NL) and eight hyperlipidaemic (HL) men with documented CAD, and compared them to 27 symptom-free controls: 17 NL men (healthy) and 10 NL men with entirely normal coronary arteriograms (CAD-free). In both Lp (A-I with A-II) and Lp (A-I without A-II), there were significantly fewer particles in the 9.2–11.2 nm region and more in the 7.0–8.2 nm region. Thus the spectrum of HDL particle sizes in patients with CAD tended to be smaller. This was observed in both NL and HL CAD patients with HDLC levels between 31 and 57 mg/dl (mean 42 ± 7 mg/dl). When controls and patients were compared, abnormalities in HDL and HDL2 levels were not signifi-cantly more frequent (twofold) among CAD patients than among controls. However, an increased fraction of 7.0–8.2 nm particles and a reduced fraction of 9.2–11.2 nm particles were 5–11 times more frequent among CAD patients ($p < 0.05$–0.0001). Thus, in two separate apo-specific HDL sub-populations, the presence of CAD was found to be more strongly associated with abnormalities in particle size than with low HDLC levels.

HDL AND OXIDATION OF LDLC

What follows is a brief summary of observations supporting the idea that oxidatively modified LDL (ox-LDL) play an important role in several atherogenic processes and that HDL, as well as certain known antioxidants, can inhibit peroxidation of LDL and cell damage by ox-LDL. First, macrophages, the principal cells of the initiating stages of atherogenesis[24,25] do not internalize unmodified LDL at a sufficient rate to result in appreciable lipid accumulation. However, oxidized LDL[26,27] is taken up in large amounts by the cell's scavenger receptor leading to cholesterol ester accumulation[28]. Second, further research has identified other mechanisms by which modified LDL is atherogenic:

(a) macrophage interactions: ox-LDL are chemo-attractants for circulating monocytes[29]; yet they inhibit macrophage tissue motility.

(b) cytotoxicity: ox-LDL, or its soluble products, are toxic[30] to endothelial cells and SMC and may contribute to central plaque necrosis and to endothelial cell dysfunction.

For example, vasorelaxation mediated by endothelial elaboration of nitric oxide (EDRF)[31] and PDGF-B[32] are inhibited by ox-LDL.

Third, although difficult to demonstrate in plasma in humans, ox-LDL accumulates in the arterial intima *in vivo*[33,34,35]. Fourth, known antioxidants appear to protect against LDL oxidation and also against the atherogenic effects of ox-LDL[36–40]. Vitamins C and E inhibit LDL oxidation[37], and atherogenesis in Watanabe rabbits was suppressed by probucol, independent of its LDL-lowering effect[38]. Furthermore, men with CAD in the Harvard Physicians Study had 44% fewer MIs while taking β-carotene[39], which is known to prevent LDL oxidation *in vitro*[40]. Fifth, HDL itself, when incubated with LDL and with endothelial cells or copper, prevents the expected LDL oxidation[41]. Finally, HDL appears to protect a lymphoblastoid cell line against the expected cytotoxicity from oxidized LDL[42].

The composite evidence supports the idea that oxidatively, or even minimally[29], modified LDL are potentially important contributors to atherogenesis. HDL has been shown to be an antioxidant and a cytoprotectant; it thus appears reasonable to hypothesize that the inverse association of HDLC with atherosclerotic events is mediated

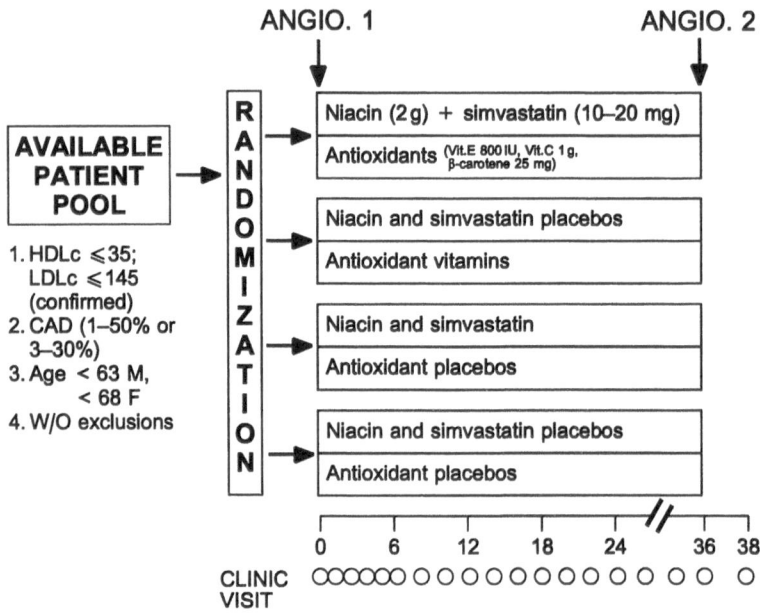

Fig. 2. Protocol diagram for the HDL Atherosclerosis Treatment Study. $n = 160$ men and women.

by these mechanisms and further that, by raising HDL or by supplementing the plasma with naturally occurring antioxidants, these atherogenic processes can be halted.

HDL ATHEROSCLEROSIS TREATMENT STUDY

No clinical or angiographic trials have ever been conducted in patients whose principal risk factor is low HDLC ($\leqslant 35$ mg/dl). We have proposed and been granted funding for just such a study, a 5 year arteriographic trial in 180 patients who should contribute 160 follow-up angiograms during the study period. The trial design is outlined in Figure 2. The patients will be men below 63 years of age and women below 68 with at least one 50% stenosis or three coronary lesions that obstruct at least 30% of the vessel lumen. They will have an HDLC of $\leqslant 35$ mg/dl and an LDLC of $\leqslant 145$ mg/dl, criteria that define a group of

Table 2. Pilot studies of niacin ± lovastatin

	Screen	Baseline	4 months
Niacin dose	–	–	1.72 g/day
Compliance	–	–	88%
Lovastatin dose	–	–	26.6 mg/day
Compliance	–	–	94%
Total cholesterol (mg/dl)	172	187 ± 24	132 ± 32
Triglycerides (mg/dl)	168	145 ± 47	92 ± 42
HDLC (mg/dl)	29	33 ± 5	42 ± 8
LDLC (mg/dl)	109	125 ± 19	72 ± 25
LDL/HDL	3.83	3.88 ± 0.71	1.84 ± 0.56
apoβ (mg/dl)	103	103 ± 14	64 ± 12
Glucose (mg/dl)	–	97 ± 15	102 ± 13
SGOT (U/L)	–	19 ± 4.0	21 ± 5.0

patients in whom HDLC seems to be the most important risk factor and for whom the original NCEP guidelines make no recommendations except 'consider diet'.

We selected the treatment on the basis of a 4-month pilot trial of niacin (0.5 g qid) together with lovastatin (20 mg qid) in 25 patients whose HDLC and LDLC met the requirements of our proposed study. Table 2 shows the results of this pilot trial. They show that this combination is well tolerated and that it produces a very substantial fall in the ratio of total to HDLC. In our arteriographic trial patients will be allocated, at random, to one of four treatment groups:

- Niacin (500 mg qid–or 1000 mg bid, as tolerated) plus simvastatin (20 mg qds), plus antioxidants (vitamin C [500 mg bid] natural vitamin E [400 IU bid] and β-carotene [12.5 mg bid])

- Niacin plus simvastatin plus antioxidant placebo

- Antioxidants plus placebo niacin and simvastatin

- Placebos for all drugs

If LDLC in patients on simvastatin and niacin remains above 90 mg/dl we will increase the dose of simvastatin to 30 mg qds. Conversely, if LDLC falls below 60 mg/dl we will reduce the dose to 10 qds.

All the patients will be given advice on modifying their lifestyle in ways that tend to elevate HDLC. They will be advised to increase their consumption of monounsaturated fatty acids[43,44], reduce their weight, exercise moderately and, where appropriate, stop smoking. Post-menopausal women will be given oestrogen replacement unless oestrogens are contraindicated. We will also advise the patients' physicians to switch from diuretics and β-blockers to drugs like the ACE inhibitors, α-blockers or calcium antagonists that have less effect on plasma lipids.

The primary endpoint of the study will be the mean change in the severity of proximal stenosis, averaged per patient among the most acute narrowing found in each of the nine proximal coronary segments as measured by quantitative arteriography[11]. This is a particularly robust indicator of disease change in relatively small populations. Additional quantitative endpoints will include the average per-patient change in minimum lesion diameter averaged over the same nine proximal segments. We will also record the appearance of new lesions. Differences in the rate of regression or progression according to the severity of the lesions at baseline or levels of lipoprotein lipids or antioxidants[45-48] could provide new information on the mechanisms of atherogenesis and the effects of treatment.

Lesion severity will be assessed by selective coronary arteriography (performed at baseline and repeated 3 years later) and intravascular ultrasound[59]. The ultrasound examinations (at baseline and after 2.5 years), made with a 2.9 Fr (0.95 mm) IVUS catheter and a 30 MHz transducer, will focus on apparently normal arterial segments and on mild to moderate lesions ($\leqslant$ 50% stenosis).

Our sample size will allow us to detect a treatment difference, in terms of our primary endpoint, of 3% with a between-patient variance of 4% at the 5% level of significance. We conservatively estimate that 35% of the lipid-untreated control group will have clinical events, as will 10% of the niacin–simvastatin group. With 160 patients the power to resolve the difference in clinical event rate between the two groups will be slightly less than 90%.

Acknowledgements

We thank Mr Robert Kelly for preparing this manuscript.

Supported in part by an NIH Grant from the U.S. Public Health Service R01 HL 49546-01A1, and in part by a grant from the John L. Locke, Jr. Charitable Trust, Seattle, WA.

References

1. Gordon T, Castelli W, Hjortland MC, Kannel WB, Dawber TR. High density lipoprotein as a protective factor against coronary heart disease: the Framingham study. Am J Med. 1977;62:707–14.
2. Gordon DJ, Probstfield JL, Garrison RJ, et al. High-density lipoprotein cholesterol and cardiovascular disease: four prospective studies. Circulation. 1989;79:8–15.
3. Castelli WP, Garrison RJ, Wilson PEF, Abbott RD, Kalousdian S, Kannel WB. Incidence of coronary heart disease and lipoprotein levels: the Framingham study. JAMA. 1986;256:2835–8.
4. Heiss G, Johnson NJ, Reiland S, Davie CE, Tyroler HA. The epidemiology of plasma high-density lipoprotein cholesterol levels: the Lipid Research Clinics Prevalence Study: Summary. Circulation. 1980;62(Suppl IV):IV-116–IV-136.
5. The Lipid Research Clinics Program. The Lipid Research Clinics Coronary Primary Prevention Trial Results: I. Reduction in incidence of coronary heart disease. JAMA. 1984;251:351–64.
6. Watkins LO, Neaton JD, Kuller LH (for the MRFIT Research Group). Radical differences in high-density lipoprotein cholesterol and coronary heart disease incidence in the Usual-Care group of the Multiple Risk Factor Intervention Trial. Am J Cardiol. 1986;57:538–45.
7. Stampfer MJ, Sacks FM, Salvini S, Willett WC, Hennekens CH. A prospective study of cholesterol, apoliproproteins, and the risk of myocardial infarction. N Engl J Med. 1991;325:373–81.
8. Johansson J. Carlson LA, Landiu C, Hamsten A. High density lipoproteins and coronary atherosclerosis: A strong inverse relation with the largest particles is confined to normotriglyceridemic patients. Arterioscler Thromb. 1991;11:174–82.
9. Blankenhorn DH, Johnson RL, Mack WJ, Zein HA, Vaolas LI. The influence of diet on the appearance of new lesions in human coronary arteries. JAMA. 1990;263:1646–51.
10. Phillips NR, Waters D, Havel RJ. Plasma lipoproteins and progression of coronary artery disease evaluated by angiography and clinical events. Circulation. 1993;88:2762–70.
11. Brown BG, Albers JJ, Fisher LD, et al. Regression of coronary artery disease as a result of intensive lipid-lowering therapy in men with high levels of apoliproprotein B. N Engl J Med. 1990;323:1289–98.
12. Stewart BF, Brown B, Zhao X-Q, et al. Benefits of lipid-lowering therapy in men with elevated apolipoprotein B are not confined to those with very high low density lipoprotein cholesterol. JACC. 1994;23:899–906.
13. Le NA, Ginsberg HN. Heterogeneity of apolipoprotein A-I turnover in subjects with reduced concentrations of plasma high density lipoprotein cholesterol. Metabolism. 1988;37:614–17.
14. Schaefer EJ, Ordovas JM, Law SW, et al. Familial apolipoprotein A-I and C-III deficiency. Variant II. J Lipid Res. 1985;26:1089–101.
15. Miller NE. Raising high density lipoprotein cholesterol. The biochemical pharmacology of reverse cholesterol transport. Biochem Pharmacol. 1990;40:403–10.
16. Schaefer EJ. Clinical, biochemical, and genetic features in familial disorders or high density lipoprotein deficiency. Arteriosclerosis. 1984;4:303–22.
17. Paigen B, Nesbitt MN, Mitchell D, Albee D, LeBouef RC. Ath-2, a second gene determining atherosclerosis susceptibility and high density lipoprotein levels in mice. Genetics. 1989;122:163–8.

18. Walsh A, Ito Y, Breslow JL. High levels of human apoliproprotein A-I in transgenic mice result in increased plasma levels of small high density lipoprotein (HDL) particles comparable to human. J Biol Chem. 1989;264:6488–92.
19. Rubin EM, Krauss RM, Spangler EA, Verstuyft JG, Clift SM. Inhibition of early atherogenesis in transgenic mice by human apolipoprotein A-I. Nature. 1991;353:265–7.
20. Warden CH, Medrick CC Qiao JH, Castellani LW, Lkusis AJ. Atherosclerosis in transgenic mice over-expressing apolipoprotein A-II. Science. 1993;261:469–71.
21. Maher VMG, Brown BG, Zhao X-Q, Cheung M, Marcovina SM, Albers JJ. Contrasting effects of apoproteins A-I and A-II on coronary artery disease change in men during 25 years of lipid-lowering therapy (abstract). JACC. 1994;23(Suppl A):100A.
22. Cheung MC, Albers JJ. Characterization of lipoprotein particles isolated by immunoaffinity chromatography. Particles containing AI and AII and particles containing AI but not AII. J Biol Chem. 1984;259:12201–9.
23. Cheung MC, Brown BG, Wolf AC, Albers JJ. Altered particle size distribution of apolipoprotein A1 containing lipoproteins in subjects with coronary artery disease. J Lipid Res. 1991;32:383–94.
24. Schaffner T, Taylor K, Bartucci EJ, et al. Arterial foam cells with distinctive immunomorphologic and histochemical features of macrophages. Am J Pathol. 1980;100:57–80.
25. Gerrity RG. The role of monocyte in atherogenesis. I. Transition of blood-borne monocytes into foam cells in fatty lesions. Am J Pathol. 1981;103:181–90.
26. Steinbrecher UP, Parthasarathy S, Leake DS, Witztum JL, Steinberg D. Modification of low density lipoprotein by endothelial cells involves lipid peroxidation and degradation of low density lipoprotein phospholipids. Proc Natl Acad Sci USA. 1984;81:3883–7.
27. Heinecke JW, Baker L, Rosen L, Chait A. Superoxide-mediated modification of low density lipoprotein by arterial smooth muscle cells. J Clin Invest. 1986;77:757–61.
28. Goldstein JL, How UK, Basu SK, Brown MS. Binding site on macrophages that mediates uptake and degradation of acelylated low density lipoprotein, producing massive cholesterol deposition. Proc Natl Acad Sci USA. 1979;76:333–7.
29. Berliner JA, Territo MC, Sevanian A, et al. Minimally modified LDL stimulates monocyte endothelial interactions. J Clin Invest. 1990;85:1260–6.
30. Hessler JR, Morel DW, Lewis LJ, Chisolm GM. Lipoprotein oxidation and lipoprotein-induced cytotoxicity. Arteriosclerosis. 1983;3:215–22.
31. Kugiyama K, Kerns SA, Morrisett JD, Roberts R, Henry PD. Impairment of endothelium-dependent arterial relaxation by lysolecithin in modified low-density lipoproteins. Nature. 1990;233:160–2.
32. Fox PL, Chisolm GM, DiCorleto PE. Lipoprotein-mediated inhibition of endothelial cell production of platelet-derived growth factor-like protein depends on free radical lipid peroxidation. J Biol Chem. 1987;262:6026–54.
33. Yla-Herttuala S, Palinski W, Rosenfeld ME, et al. Evidence for the presence of oxidatively modified low density lipoprotein in atherosclerotic lesions of rabbit and man. J Clin Invest. 1989;84:1086–95.
34. Palanski W, Rosenfeld ME, Yla-Herttuala S, et al. Low density lipoprotein undergoes oxidative modification in vivo. Proc Natl Acad Sci USA. 1989;86:1372–6.
35. Haberland M, Fong D, Cheng L. Malondialdehyde-altered protein occurs in atheroma of Watanabe heritable hyperlipidemic rabbits. Science. 1988;24:215–18.

36. Jialal I, Norkus EP, Cristol LS, Grundy SM. Inhibition of LDL oxidation by beta-carotene (abstract). Circulation. 1991;84(Suppl II):II-449.
37. Jialal I, Grundy SM. Preservation of endogenous antioxidants in low density lipoprotein by ascorbate but not probucol during oxidative modification. J Clin Invest. 1991;87:597–601.
38. Carew TE, Schwenke DC, Steinberg D. Antiatherogenic effect of probucol unrelated to its hypocholesterolemic effect: Evidence that antioxidants in vivo can selectively inhibit low density lipoprotein degradation in macrophage-rich fatty streaks and slow the progression of atherosclerosis in the Watanabe heritable hyperlipidemic rabbit. Proc Natl Acad Sci USA. 1987;84:7725–9.
39. Gaziano JM, Manson JE, Ridker PM, Buring JE, Hennekens CH. Beta-carotene therapy for chronic stable angina (abstract). Circulation. 1990;84(Suppl III):III-201.
40. Jialal I, Norkus EP, Cristol LS, Grundy SM. Inhibition of LDL oxidation by beta-carotene (abstract). Circulation. 1991;84(Suppl II):II-449.
41. Parthasarathy S, Barnett J, Fong LG. High-density lipoprotein inhibits the oxidative modification of low-density lipoprotein. Biochem Biophys Acta. 1990:1044:275–83.
42. Douste-Blaxy L, N'egre-Salvayre A, Lopex M, Salvayre R. The cytotoxicity of oxidized lipoproteins. Bull Acad Natl Med. 1989;173:903–10.
43. Mattson FH. A changing role for dietary monounsaturated fatty acids. J Am Diet Assoc. 1989;89:387–91.
44. Ginsberg HN, Barr SL, Gilbert A, et al. Reduction of plasma cholesterol levels in normal men on an American Heart Association Step I diet or a Step I diet with added monounsaturated fat. N Engl J Med. 1990;322:574–9.
45. Marcovina SM, Albers JJ, Dati F, Ledue TB, Ritchie RF. International Federation of Clinical Chemistry standardization project for measurements of apolipropro-teins A-I and B. Clin Chem. 1991;37:1676–82.
46. Albers JJ, Segrest JP, editors. Enzymatic methods for quantification of lipoprotein lipids. In: Methods in enzymology, Vol. 129, Plasma lipoproteins, Part B, Characterization cell biology, and metabolism. New York: Academic Press, Inc.; 1986:101–23.
47. Albers JJ. Beta quantification procedures: Lipid resources clinical program: Vol. 1 (Lipids and lipoproteins). Washington, D.C.: Government (DHEW) Publication Number NIH 75-628; 1974.
48. Warnick GR, Benderson J, Albers JJ, et al. Dextran sulfate-Mg^{2+} precipitation procedure for quantification of high-density lipoprotein cholesterol. Clin Chem. 1982;28:1379–88.
49. Bachorik PS, Albers JJ. Precipitation methods for quantification of lipoproteins In: Albers JJ, Segrest JP, editors. Methods in enzymology. Vol. 129, Plasma lipoproteins, Part B, Characterization, cell biology, and metabolism. New York: Academic Press, Inc.; 1986:78-100.
50. Warnick GR, Benderson J, Albers JJ, et al. Dextran sulfate-Mg^{2+} precipitation procedure for quantification of high-density lipoprotein cholesterol. Clin Chem. 1982;28:1379-88.
51. Marcovina SM, Albers JJ. International Federation of Clinical Chemistry study on the standardization of apolipoproteins A-I and B. Curr Opin Lipid. 1991;2:355–61.
52. Marcovina SM, Albers JJ, Jenderson LO, Hannon WH. Standardization project for measurements of apolipoproteins A-I and B. III. Comparability of Apo A-I

41

values by the use of common reference material. Clin Chem. [Manuscript submitted].

53. Albers JJ, Marcovina SM, Lodge MS. Problems related to the immunochemical determination of Lp(a). Clin Chem. 1990;36:2019–26.

54. Bierrei JG, et al. Simultaneous determination of α-tocopherol and retinol in plasma or red cells by high performance liquid chromatography. Am J Clin Nutr. 1979;32:2143–9.

55. Margolis SA, David TP. Stabilization of ascorbic acid in human plasma, and its liquid-chromatographic measurement. Clin Chem. 1988;32:2217–23.

56. Tulley RT. New enzymatic method for vitamin C in plasma on CX5. Clin Chem. 1992;38:1070.

57. Craft NE, Wise SA. Optimization of an isocratic high-performance liquid chromatographic separation of carotenoids. J Chromatogr. 1992;589:171–6.

58. Esterbauer H, Streigl G, Puhl H. Continuous monitoring of in vitro oxidation of human LDL. Free Radic Res Commun. 1989;6:67–75.

59. Fitzgerald PJ, St Goar FG, Conolly RJ, et al. Intravascular ultrasound imaging of coronary arteries: is three layers the norm? Circulation. 1992;86:154–8.

5

Intracellular cholesterol transport

U. SEEDORF, P. BRYSCH, T. ENGEL, S. SCHEEK,
M. RAABE, M. FOBKER, T. SZYPERSKI, K. WÜTHRICH,
N. MAEDA and G. ASSMANN

Intracellular trafficking of cholesterol and various other sterols is important for cholesterol homeostasis of cells and the entire organism. Understanding the mechanisms involved in regulated, target-specific intracellular cholesterol transport is of great impact for understanding the pathogenesis of atherosclerosis and a number of inherited lipid storage disorders, such as Niemann–Pick disease (type C), Zellweger disease and Tangier disease. Since, in humans, only the liver contains the enzymes necessary for cholesterol degradation, all other tissues in the body have to export excess cholesterol to this organ in a pathway called reverse cholesterol transport. It is obvious that this pathway represents an important mechanism protecting cells and tissues from cholesterol overloading, a phenomenon observed in cells of the arterial wall during atherogenesis. The initial steps consisting of a target-specific flux of cholesterol from intracellular pools to the plasma membrane are only poorly understood at present. It is generally accepted that intracellular trafficking of cholesterol and other sterols is not mediated by non-specific diffusion but requires target-specific transport mechanisms. Earlier studies performed in our and other laboratories indicated that the bulk flow of *de-novo* synthesized cholesterol from the endoplasmic reticulum to the plasma membrane is a fast, energy-requiring, vesicular process that proceeds independently of the secretory protein pathway[1]. Specific transport mechanisms have also been suggested for the transfer of cholesterol from the membranes of secondary lysosomes to the endoplasmic reticulum, the intracellular site of cholesterol esterification catalysed by the enzyme acyl-CoA cholesterol acyl transferase (ACAT), and the delivery of sterols to mitochondria and peroxisomes[2]. The latter pathways are primarily required for the synthesis of pregnenolone and bile acids. The precise mechanisms have, however, not been established.

Three mechanistic models explaining target-specific intracellular sterol transport have been suggested: transport via specialized lipid-rich vesicles, intracellular lipoprotein-like particles, and sterol carrier proteins. The sequential action of several of these mechanisms is certainly also possible. Sterol transport via soluble carrier proteins is a very attractive hypothesis. The proteins could harbour signals mediating target-specificity and, at the same time, shield the lipophilic transport substrates from the aqueous phase. The best-known candidate for a sterol carrier is sterol carrier protein 2 (SCP2). SCP2, also known as the non-specific lipid transfer protein, promotes the exchange of a wide variety of lipids and sterols between membranes *in vitro*[3]. In addition, the protein activates the enzymatic conversion of 7-DHC to cholesterol by liver microsomes[4]. It also stimulates the acyl-CoA cholesterol acyltransferase-mediated esterification of intracellular cholesterol[5] and the introduction of the less-polar substrates in bile acid biosynthesis to the membrane-bound enzymes *in vitro*[6]. Moreover, the protein may be required for the intracellular transfer of cholesterol needed for pregnenolone synthesis in adrenals[7] and ovaries[8]. On the other hand, purified SCP2 does not contain any bound lipid[9], and a stable association between SCP2 and phospholipids or cholesterol could not be demonstrated[10]. Therefore, it was proposed that the protein either binds lipids with low affinity[11] or does not function as a typical binding protein, but facilitates lipid exchange between membranes by other means[12]. In view of the high degree of specificity required for the function of intracellular sterol transport, the structural simplicity of SCP2, deduced from its primary sequence[13], seems at least to be surprising.

To evaluate the hypothesis that SCP2 functions as an intracellular sterol carrier, we employed methods of current molecular biology. We first cloned and sequenced SCP2-encoding cDNAs from the rat[14], mouse[15], and human (Seedorf, unpublished). These studies indicated that mammalian SCP2 is synthesized as a 143 amino-acid precursor that is processed to the 123 amino-acid mature SCP2. In addition, SCP2-related transcripts encoding larger proteins which are identical at their C-terminal domains with pre-SCP2 are present in the livers of all mammalian species studied. The complete cDNA encoding one of these proteins has an open reading frame of 547 codons representing an extension of 404 codons at the initiator methionine of pre-SCP2. The

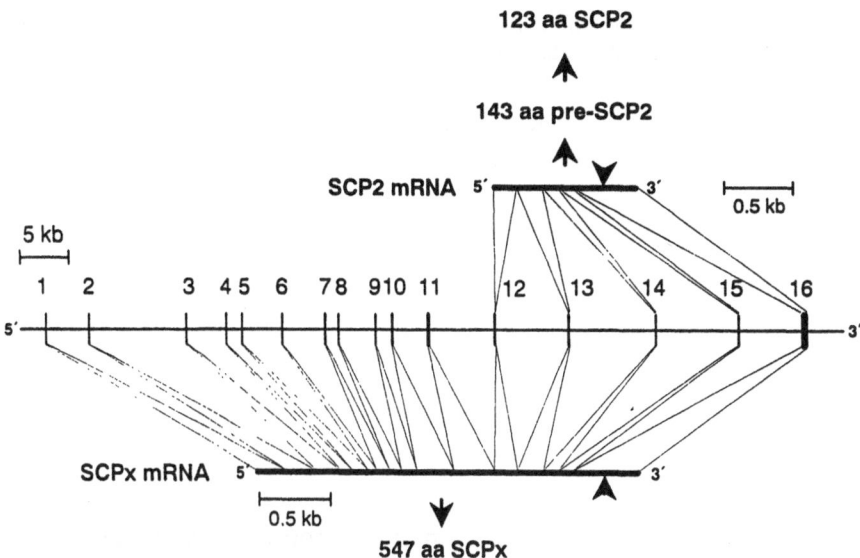

Fig. 1. Structure of the murine SCP2/SCPx gene and alternative splicing and/or transcription initiation pathways

open reading frame was predicted to encode a previously undescribed fusion protein containing a 143 amino-acid C-terminal lipid transfer domain and a 404 amino-acid N-terminal domain with unknown biochemical activity or function. Since the fact that SCP2 is completely contained within this sequence suggested possible sterol carrier activity we assigned the predicted protein the preliminary name sterol carrier protein x (SCPx)[14].

Most recent work in our laboratory focused on the mouse model. As shown in Figure 1, SCP2 and SCPx are encoded by a single gene consisting of 16 exons spanning almost 100 kb, located on the murine chromosome 3 or 4. SCP2 and SCPx transcripts are produced by alternative splicing and/or alternative transcription initiation. The coding information of exons 1–16 is used to generate SCPx, whereas exons 12–16 are spliced to create the SCP2 transcript. Further transcript heterogeneity results from alternative polyadenylation of the two types of transcripts[15]. In addition we have isolated and characterized two SCP2-related pseudogenes, SCP2-ps1 and SCP2-ps2, both of which have similar structures lacking introns and are not transcribed[15] (Seedorf and Raabe, unpublished). A preliminary evaluation of our data

Table 1. Specific activities of SCPx-547 determined with various 3-ketoacyl-CoA substrates. For experimental details see ref. 16

Acyl-CoA substrate	Acyl-chain length	V_{max} (U/mg)
Acetoacetyl-CoA	C4:0	2.5
3-Ketohexanoyl-CoA	C6:0	55.4
3-Ketooctanoyl-CoA	C8:0	120
3-Ketodecanoyl-CoA	C10:0	48.9
3-Ketoundecanoyl-CoA	C11:0	53.3
3-Ketomyristoyl-CoA	C14:0	35.3
3-Ketopalmitoyl-CoA	C16:0	30.6
3-Ketostearoyl-CoA	C18:0	26.7
3-Ketooleoyl-CoA	C18:1	33.3

suggests that the overall organization of the mouse and human genes is very similar.

To elucidate possible biological functions of SCPx, we expressed the entire rat SCPx (SCPx-547) and a peptide consisting of the thiolase-like SCPx-specific domain (residues 1–383, SCPx-383) in *E. coli*. Subcellular fractionation followed by Western blotting analysis with antibodies against SCPx-383, which did not cross-react with SCP2, revealed that SCPx is primarily localized within peroxisomes[16]. This result was confirmed by immunocytochemistry revealing SCPx-383 epitopes within the matrix of organelles containing an electron-dense lattice-like structure, characteristic for peroxisomes. In contrast, relatively little SCP2 was detected in this organelle, suggesting that this protein has a more widespread intracellular localization[16].

Since the sequence of the N-terminal 400 amino acids of SCPx is known to be vaguely related to acetoacetyl-CoA and 3-ketoacyl-CoA thiolases, we further investigated whether SCPx-547 has thiolase activity if tested in an *in vitro* β-oxidation system[16]. As shown in Table 1, SCPx-547 efficiently catalyses the thiolytic cleavage of a wide variety of 3-ketoacyl-CoA substrates. The highest specific activity was obtained with 3-ketooctanoyl-CoA (V_{max} = 120 U/mg). Acyl chain lengths above or below 8 carbon atoms resulted in a gradual decrease in specific activity. The enzyme is a very poor catalyst of the thiolytic cleavage of acetoacetyl-CoA (specific activity 2.5 U/mg). The activities obtained with the unsaturated substrate 3-ketooleoyl-CoA (C18:1) and the saturated substrate 3-ketostearoyl-CoA (C18:0) are similar (33.3 and 26.7 U/mg) (Table 1). Like all the known thiolases, the SCPx-thiolase uses a ping-pong reaction mechanism. The first partial reaction is the formation of acetyl-CoA and an $acyl_{(n-2)}$-S-enzyme, whereas in the second partial reaction the $acyl_{(n-2)}$ moiety is transferred to CoA, resulting in saturated fatty $acyl_{(n-2)}$-CoA and the free enzyme form. The apparent K_M values for CoA are 2.9 $\pm$ 0.59 and 6.3 $\pm$ 1.3 µmol/l ([3-ketooctanoyl-CoA] = 2.5 and 10 µmol/l), suggesting that the enzyme has a high affinity for CoA. The apparent K_M values of 5.4 and 7.9 µmol/l ([CoA] = 150 µmol/l) obtained for 3-ketooctanoyl CoA and 3-ketopalmitoyl-CoA point to a somewhat higher affinity for the medium than for the long acyl chain substrate[16]. The classical Michaelis–Menten kinetic relationship between substrate concentrations and initial velocities found for the medium acyl chain substrate 3-ketooctanoyl-CoA is altered to a sigmoidal curve for the long acyl chain substrate 3-ketopalmitoyl-CoA[16]. Therefore, efficient thiolytic cleavage of the long acyl chain substrate is *in vitro* dependent on relatively high substrate concentrations.

The latter finding discriminates the novel thiolase from the previously described peroxisomal 3-ketoacyl-CoA thiolase that was reported to exhibit significantly higher affinities for long than for medium acyl chain substrates[17]. Peroxisomal 3-ketoacyl-CoA thiolase was further shown to be regulated by acetyl-CoA-mediated product inhibition. It was suggested that acetyl-CoA binds to the CoA site of the enzyme as a dead-end inhibitor, resulting in strong product inhibition at acetyl-CoA concentrations as low as 30 µmol/l[17]. The SCPx thiolase shows different behaviour. Since acetyl-CoA is competitive with respect to CoA (K_I: 20.4 $\pm$ 2.0 µmol/l) and non-competitive with respect to 3-ketooctanoyl-CoA (K_I: 29.0 $\pm$ 5.5 µmol/l), acetyl-CoA reacts with the enzyme classically as the first product in the ping-pong reaction mechanism[16].

Since SCPx contains the SCP2-identical domain at its C-terminus, we also investigated whether the protein has the same ability to stimulate the microsomal conversion of 7-DHC to cholesterol as SCP2 (known as sterol carrier activity). We found that SCPx stimulates this *in-vitro* reaction, although to a somewhat lower extent than SCP2. To exclude a direct stimulatory effect of SCPx on microsomal sterol Δ^7-reductase, the enzyme catalysing the reaction, we also measured the transfer of 7-DHC from small unilamellar vesicles to *Bacillus megaterium* protoplasts directly. Using this assay we could show that SCPx-547 transfers 16.3

nmol/(nmol × h) representing 53% of the value for SCP2 (30.6 nmol/(nmol × h)). Moreover, SCPx has almost the same sterol transfer activity as an artificial fusion protein constructed between glutathione-S-transferase and SCP2 (GST-SCP2), suggesting that the N-terminal thiolase-like domain has no specific influence on the transfer activity of SCPx-547. Another well-documented activity of SCP2 is the transfer of phosphatidylcholine (PC) from donor small unilamellar vesicles to *Bacillus megaterium* protoplasts[18]. We found that SCPx transfers 64 nmol PC/(nmol × h) representing 34% of the molar activity of SCP2 (189 nmol/(nmol × h)).

What is the structural basis of SCP2- and SCPx-mediated sterol and phospholipid transfer? We addressed this question by site-directed mutagenesis of recombinant human SCP2 combined with three-dimensional nuclear magnetic resonance spectroscopy with [15-N]-labelled human SCP2[18,19]. Three α-helices comprising the polypeptide segments of residues 9–22, 25–30 and 100–102 were identified by sequential and medium-range nuclear Overhauser effects (NOE). The analysis of long-range backbone–backbone NOEs further revealed a five-stranded β-sheet including the residues 33–41, 47–54, 60–62, 71–76 and 100–102. Figure 2 shows the ribbon drawings of residues 8–76 and 99–103 of the optimized conformer omitting helix C, since its precise arrangement has not yet been elucidated. SCP2 consists of a very unusual α–β-tertiary fold. No near identity was found with any of the protein folding types which are known to exist. The central feature of the molecular architecture consists of the central β-sheet. The first three strands are arranged in an antiparallel fashion; the polypeptide chain then crosses over this sheet in right-handed sense so that the fourth strand is added parallel to the first one. The fifth strand runs antiparallel to the fourth one, so that the total topology is +1, +1, –3x, –1. The β-sheet forms a flat, nearly oval structure, which is surrounded by three amphipatic α-helices (Figure 2). The hydrophobic surface of the β-sheet faces the hydrophobic surface of the amphipatic helix A. Schematically, the whole structure resembles an amphipatic plate or dish consisting of a hydrophilic outer part and an essentially hydrophobic inner part. A preliminary interpretation of this structure implies that SCP2 has no well-defined lipid-binding site, as there is, for example, in the fatty acid binding protein (FABP) which was shown to contain a hydrophobic pocket within its globular structure. Currently, we assume that the hydrophobic cleft created between helix A and the hydrophobic surface

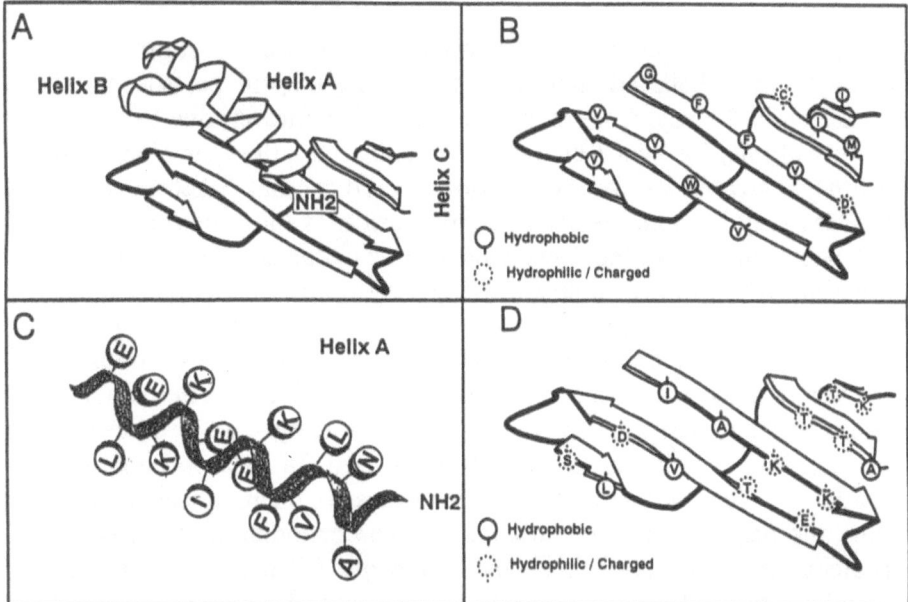

Fig. 2. Three-dimensional polypeptide backbone fold of human SCP2. Ribbon drawing generated with program Molscript of residues 8–76 and 99–103 of the optimal DIANA conformer without helix C (**A**). Amphipaticity of the central five-stranded β-sheet. Amino-acid side chains exposed to the top (**B**) and to the bottom (**D**). Amphipaticity of helix A (**C**). For methodological details see ref. 19

of the β-sheet interacts in a rather non-specific fashion with lipids. This view is clearly supported by results obtained by *site-directed* mutagenesis[18]. Mutations which interfere with helix A or the integrity of the central β-sheet lead to drastic inactivation of SCP2-mediated sterol and phospholipid transfer. In contrast, mutations outside this structure, or mutations which would have no effect on this structure, have almost no effect on SCP2 activity.

The *in-vivo-function* of the novel peroxisomal 3-ketoacyl-CoA thiolase with intrinsic *in-vitro* sterol carrier and PC transfer activity remains to be elucidated. Since another peroxisomal 3-ketoacyl-CoA thiolase has been known for more than 10 years, the idea that this enzyme which exists in two closely related isoforms is completely sufficient to catalyse the thiolytic cleavage of all 3-ketoacyl-CoA substrates occurring in peroxisomal β-oxidation *in vivo* has to be re-evaluated[20]. We are currently following two working hypotheses. One major function discriminating peroxisomal from mitochondrial β-oxidation is to supply acetyl-CoA for anabolic reactions when the cells are well supplied with energy[21]. It is believed that the rate-limiting step in peroxisomal β-oxidation is the acyl-CoA oxidase reaction[22]. However, due to its high relative affinity for long 3-ketoacyl-CoA substrates, thiolysis of medium-chain substrates by the conventional peroxisomal 3-ketoacyl-CoA thiolase may become inefficient at high levels of long-chain substrates (i.e. postprandially in the liver). Under these circumstances one possible function of the novel thiolase activity may be to preferentially act on medium 3-ketoacyl-CoA substrates, thus preventing their thiolytic cleavage from becoming rate-limiting. Recent studies have confirmed the assumption that peroxisomes contain all the enzymes necessary for cholesterol synthesis. It is further known that acetyl-CoA produced via peroxisomal β-oxidation is preferentially used for *de-novo* cholesterol synthesis[23], suggesting that the two pathways are interconnected. There-fore, the gene fusion event between a gene encoding a sterol carrier protein and a gene encoding a medium-chain 3-ketoacyl-CoA thiolase may have been of selective advantage. The second possibility would be that, despite the fact that medium chain 3-ketoacyl-CoAs are efficiently cleaved by the SCPx thiolase *in vitro*, they are not the real substrates *in vivo*. A major function of peroxisomal β-oxidation is the oxidative degradation of xenobiotics and the cholesterol side-chain. Since it cannot be excluded at present that the novel SCP2/3-ketoacyl-CoA thiolase participates in these pathways *in vivo*, we are currently further investigating the substrate specificity of the novel enzyme.

Another approach that can be used in order to evaluate these hypotheses is to generate mice lacking the SCPx gene function. To proceed with this goal we constructed a gene targeting vector. An approximately 7 kb EcoRI fragment containing exon 14 of the murine SCP2/SCPx gene and the flanking intron regions was isolated from a genomic λ-clone and subcloned in the vector pBluescript. The con-tinuity of exon 14 was then disrupted by inserting a neo[R]-gene and the resulting DNA fragment was cloned in the vector pPNT (Fig. 3). Subsequently, this vector was used in collaboration with Dr Maeda (UNC at Chapel Hill) to transfect E14TG2a mouse embryonic stem cells. Selection with G418 and gancyclovir led to the isolation of 182 resistant clones. Southern blotting analyses revealed two clones in which homologous recombination had occurred between the vector and the endogenous exon 14 region of the SCP2/SCPx gene. These clones were subsequently used to generate chimeric mice which were then crossed

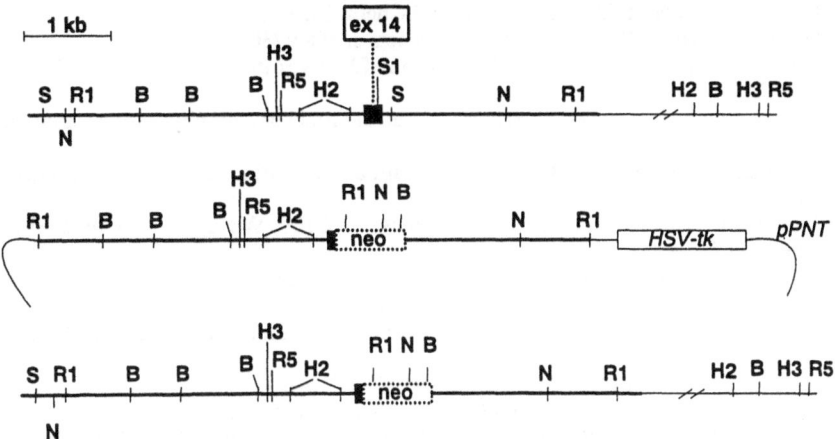

Fig. 3. Restriction nuclease map of the exon 14 region of the murine SCP2/SCPx gene (top). Structure of the gene replacement vector constructed for disruption of exon 14 (middle). Restriction nuclease map of the exon 14 region as determined after homologous recombination had occurred in clones 20 and 110. S: Spe1, N: Nco1, R1: EcoR1, B: BamH1, H3: Hind3, R5: EcoR5, H2: Hind2, S1: Sal1

with C57BL/6 mice. We identified several transmitters and are currently generating a strain of mice deficient in SCP2 and SCPx. We hope that the phenotypic characterization of these mice will help us to further understand the roles of the two sterol carrier proteins in sterol trafficking and sterol metabolism.

Acknowledgements

This work was supported by the Deutsche Forschungsgemeinschaft (grants Se 459/2-1 and Se 459/2-2), the Land Nordrhein Westfalen, and grants from the Boehringer-Ingelheim Fonds and Bristol Myers Squibb.

References

1. Seedorf U, Fobker M, Assmann G. Circulation. 1992;86(Suppl.I):549.
2. Liscum L, Dahl NK. J Lipid Res. 1992;33:1239–54.
3. Reinhart MP. Experientia. 1990;46:599–611.
4. Noland BJ, Arebalo RE, Hansbury E, Scallen TJ. J Biol Chem. 1980;255:4282–9.

5. Gavey KL, Noland BJ, Scallen TJ. J Biol Chem. 1981;256:2993–9.
6. Seltman H, Diven W, Rizk M, et al. Biochem J. 1985;230:19–24.
7. Chanderbhan R, Noland BJ, Scallen TJ, Vahouny GV. J Biol Chem. 1982;257:8928–34.
8. Chanderbhan R, Tanaka T, Strauss JF, et al. Biochem Biophys Res Commun. 1983;117:702–9.
9. Chanderbhan R, Noland BJ, Scallen TJ, Vahouny G. J Biol Chem. 1982;257:8928–34.
10. Van Amerongen A, Teerlink T, Van Heusden GPH, Wirtz KWA. Chem Phys Lipids. 1985;38:195–204.
11. Schroeder F, Butko P, Nemecz G, Scallen TJ. J Biol Chem. 1990;265:151–7.
12. Wirtz KWA, Gadella Jr TWJ. Experientia. 1990;46:592–9.
13. Pastuszyn A, Noland BJ, Bazan JF, Fletterick RJ. J Biol Chem. 1987;262:13219–27.
14. Seedorf U, Assmann G. J Biol Chem. 1991;266:630–6.
15. Seedorf U, Raabe M, Assmann G. Gene. 1993;123:165–72.
16. Seedorf U, Brysch P, Engel T, Schrage K, Assmann G. J Biol Chem. 1994;269:21277–83.
17. Miyazawa S, Furuta S, Osumi T, Hashimoto T, Ui N. J Biochem (Tokyo). 1981;90:511–19.
18. Seedorf U, Scheek S, Engel T, Steif C, Hinz HJ, Assmann G. J Biol Chem. 1994;269:2613–18.
19. Szyperski T, Scheek S, Johansson J, Assmann G, Seedorf U, Wüthrich K. FEBS Lett. 1993;335:18–26.
20. Hijikata M, Wen JK, Osumi T, Hashimoto T. J Biol Chem. 1990;265:4600–6.
21. Leighton F, Nicovani S, Sotu U, Skorin C, Necochea C. In: Fahimi HD, Sies H, editors. Peroxisomes in biology and medicine. Heidelberg: Springer; 1987:177–88.
22. Hryb DJ, Hogg JF. Biochem Biophys Res Commun. 1979;87:1200–6.
23. Hayashi H, Miwa A. Arch Biochem Biophys. 1989;274:582–9.

6

Apolipoprotein E and Alzheimer's disease

R.W. MAHLEY

INTRODUCTION

Apolipoprotein (apo) E, a 34 000 molecular weight protein that is the product of a single gene on chromosome 19 (for review, see ref. 1), exists in three major forms. Its heterogeneity results from a single amino acid substitution at residue 112 or 158. The common isoform, apoE3, has cysteine at residue 112 and arginine at residue 158. The apoE4 isoform, which has been linked to Alzheimer's disease, differs from apoE3 only at residue 112, where it possesses arginine. The apoE2 isoform, associated with type III hyperlipoproteinaemia[1], differs from apoE3 only at residue 158, where it possesses cysteine. Apolipoproteins E3 and E4 bind normally to the low density lipoprotein (LDL) receptor, whereas apoE2 does not.

By redistributing lipids among the cells of different organs, apoE plays a critical role in lipid metabolism (for review, see ref. 1). While apoE exerts this global transport mechanism in chylomicron and very low density lipoprotein (VLDL) metabolism, it also functions in the local transport of lipids by redistributing them among cells within a tissue. Cells with excess cholesterol and other lipids may release these substances to apoE·lipid complexes or to high density lipoproteins (HDL) containing apoE, which can transport the lipids to cells requiring them for proliferation or repair. The apoE on these lipoprotein particles mediates their interaction and uptake via the LDL receptor or the LDL receptor-related protein (LRP).

A series of observations made over several years suggests a neurobiological role for apoE. First, apoE mRNA is abundant in the brain, where it is synthesized and secreted primarily by astrocytes[2-4]. (The brain is second only to the liver in the level of apoE mRNA expression.) Second, apoE-containing lipoproteins are found in the cerebrospinal fluid (CSF) and appear to play a major role in lipid transport in the central nervous system[5]. In fact, the major CSF lipoprotein is an HDL with apoE. Third, apoE plus a source of cholesterol promotes marked neurite extension in dorsal root ganglion cells in culture[6]. Fourth, apoE levels dramatically increase (about 250-fold) after peripheral nerve injury[7,8]. Apolipoprotein E appears to participate both in the scavenging of lipids generated after axon degeneration and in the redistribution of these lipids to sprouting neurites for axon regeneration, and later to Schwann cells for remyelination of the new axons[9,10].

Most recently, apoE has been implicated in Alzheimer's disease[11,12]. Apolipoprotein E is associated with the two characteristic neuropathological lesions of Alzheimer's disease – extracellular neuritic plaques representing deposits of amyloid beta (Aβ) peptide and intracellular neurofibrillary tangles representing filaments of hyperphosphorylated tau, a microtubule-associated protein (for review, see refs. 13–18). Three categories of Alzheimer's disease are early-onset familial disease (occurring before 60 years of age and linked to genes on chromosomes 21 and 14), late-onset familial disease, and sporadic late-onset disease. Both types of late-onset disease have recently been linked to chromosome 19 at the apoE locus. Other results suggest that apoE4 is directly linked to the severity of the disease in late-onset families[16]. For individuals in the late-onset families with no apoE4 allele, the risk of developing the disease was about 20%, and onset occurred at 84 years of age. Individuals with apoE4 for both alleles had a 90% risk of developing the disease, and the age of onset was approximately 68 years.

A marked overrepresentation of apoE4 occurs in patients with Alzheimer's disease[11,12]. In a normal population, apoE4 is rare, occurring in about 15% of the population. However, about 40–50% of the Alzheimer's patient group has apoE4.

Apolipoprotein E and amyloid plaque formation

Biochemically it has been shown that the Aβ peptide and apoE4 interact readily *in vitro* to form a very stable complex[19,20], whereas apoE3 displays a less avid interaction with Aβ. Morphological studies using negative staining electron microscopy revealed interesting differences in the ultrastructures of apoE·Aβ peptide complexes formed with apoE3 versus apoE4[21]. When Aβ was incubated alone, it formed characteristic flat, ribbon-like structures. However, when apoE4 and Aβ were incubated together, dense complexes composed of very long monofibrils, similar to those seen in neuritic plaques, were observed. The network of monofibrils observed in the presence of apoE4 was massive, whereas that seen in the presence of apoE3 was less extensive. When incubated with apoE3, much of the Aβ peptide appeared unreactive, many Aβ ribbon-like structures were present, and the monofibrillar complex was less dense. Similar results have recently been reported by Ma et al.[22]. Immunogold labelling demonstrated that apoE3 or apoE4 was associated with the monofibrils formed with Aβ. The apoE may have been strongly absorbed along the surface of the fibrils or incorporated within them[21].

The complex plaque formed with Aβ in the presence of apoE4 *in vivo* could impair the normal clearance process and enhance further plaque formation. In contrast, apoE3 may allow more normal clearance of Aβ and thus impair plaque formation, or at least the extent of deposition. The Aβ peptide is generated normally in nerve tissue and under most circumstances does not accumulate. Amyloid plaques may be toxic to neurons, and in this way contribute to pathogenesis.

Apolipoprotein E and neurofibrillary tangles

The neurofibrillary tangles, which are paired helical filaments of hyperphosphorylated tau (for review, see refs. 15, 17 and 18), accumulate in the cytoplasm of neurons. Tau is a microtubule-associated phosphoprotein which normally participates in microtubule assembly and stabilization; however, hyperphosphorylation impairs its ability to interact with microtubules.

It has been shown that tau interacts with apoE3 *in vitro*, but not with apoE4[23]. The interaction of apoE3 with tau may prevent tau's hyperphosphorylation, thus allowing it to function normally in stabilizing microtubular structure and function[17,23]. In the presence of apoE4, tau could become hyperphosphorylated and thus inactive, which could promote the formation of neurofibrillary tangles.

RESULTS AND DISCUSSION

In neurons, the cytoskeleton functions in neurite extension and retraction. Therefore, our studies have focused on the isoform-specific effects of apoE3 and apoE4 on neurite extension and branching. Our postulate is that apoE modulates the intracellular cytoskeletal apparatus and alters neurite extension and branching. Understanding how the various isoforms of apoE alter the cytoskeleton may shed light on the process of neurofibrillary tangle formation and suggest how apoE may modulate the remodelling of synaptic connections later in life.

Incubation of dorsal root ganglion neurons in culture with β-VLDL or cholesterol alters the neurite growth of these cells compared to that of cells grown in media alone[6]. In the presence of a source of lipid (β-VLDL or free cholesterol), neurite outgrowth is greatly enhanced, specifically due to extensive branching (with little or no neurite extension). When rabbit apoE (equivalent to human apoE3 with respect to the occurrence of cysteine at residue 112) was added to this system, however, very significant neurite extension was seen[6]. A source of cholesterol appears to enhance membrane biosynthesis, whereas the addition of rabbit apoE with a source of lipid results in long neuritic extensions and a trimming back of the branches. The elongation of neurites in cultured neurons may stimulate neurite extension, which could promote nerve regeneration or the formation of synaptic connections during neuronal remodelling.

A comparison of the effects of human apoE3 versus human apoE4 showed pronounced differential isoform-specific effects on neurite outgrowth[24]. Apolipoprotein E3 plus β-VLDL resulted in an increase in neurite extension, while apoE4 plus β-VLDL resulted in a marked decrease in both neurite branching and extension. Dorsal root ganglion neurons incubated with apoE4 plus β-VLDL displayed very short, stunted neurites[24]. This was not a toxic effect of apoE4 since replacement of the apoE4-containing media with fresh apoE4-lacking media restored the ability of the neurons to produce neuritic extensions. Furthermore, the apoE3- and apoE4-specific effects were blocked by addition of an antibody against the receptor-binding domain of apoE or reductive methylation of critical lysine residues, suggesting that the effect of apoE was receptor-mediated.

Murine neuroblastoma cells (Neuro-2a) from the central nervous system were used to compare the effects of apoE on the peripheral nervous system neurons described above with those on cortical neurons. Cells of both types respond similarly to apoE. When combined with a source of lipid, apoE3 stimulated neurite extension, whereas apoE4 inhibited it[25]. Addition of free apoE3 or apoE4 without β-VLDL had no effect on neurite outgrowth. These results further suggest that the effect of apoE on neurons requires the lipoprotein receptor-mediated uptake of apoE or a combination of apoE plus a source of lipid. Free of lipid, apoE does not bind to either the LDL receptor or the LRP.

Apolipoprotein E3 or E4 plus β-VLDL was incubated with Neuro-2a cells for 48 hours, and intracellular apoE was localized by immuno-fluorescence using confocal microscopy[25]. By optical sectioning through the neuronal cell body and neurites, apoE was visualized on the cell surface and throughout the cell. Apolipoprotein E3 accumulated in high concentration in the cell bodies around the nucleus and diffusely throughout the neurites within the intracellular compartment. Although apoE3 clearly is present intracellularly, it is not yet possible to ascertain whether it occurs within the cytoplasm, in association with the cytoskeletal elements, or within vesicles. On the other hand, apoE4 accumulated in the cell bodies and neurites to a much lesser degree; it was localized near the cell surface and to a much lesser extent within the short neurites. Although we have demonstrated that apoE3 and apoE4 in the presence of β-VLDL are taken up by the cells to a similar extent, apoE3 appears to be retained, whereas apoE4 is not.

SUMMARY

In dorsal root ganglion or neuroblastoma cells, apoE3 plus a source of lipid supports and facilitates neurite extension. Apolipoprotein E3 appears to accumulate widely in cell bodies and neurites, stabilize the cytoskeleton and support neurite elongation, and directly or indirectly modulate cytoskeletal activity. Apolipoprotein E4, on the other hand, does not appear to accumulate within neurons or to support neurite extension, and may even destabilize the cytoskeleton. Individuals with apoE4 clearly have normal neuronal development early in life. However, apoE4 may exert its detrimental effects later in life, by not allowing or supporting remodelling of synaptic connections. This effect may be important in the pathogenesis of Alzheimer's disease. Alternatively, apoE4 may contribute to Alzheimer's disease by aiding the formation of dense, complicated, possibly toxic plaques of Aβ peptide. At present, the pathway whereby apoE affects the development of Alzheimer's disease remains speculative.

Acknowledgement

This research was funded in part by NIH Program Project Grant HL41633.

References

1. Mahley RW. Apolipoprotein E: cholesterol transport protein with expanding role in cell biology. Science. 1988;240:622–30.
2. Elshourbagy NA, Liao WS, Mahley RW, Taylor JM. Apolipoprotein E mRNA is abundant in the brain and adrenals, as well as in the liver, and is present in other peripheral tissues of rats and marmosets. Proc Natl Acad Sci USA. 1985;82:203–7.
3. Boyles JK, Pitas RE, Wilson E, Mahley RW, Taylor JM. Apolipoprotein E associated with astrocytic glia of the central nervous system and with nonmyelinating glia of the peripheral nervous system. J Clin Invest. 1985;76:1501–13.
4. Pitas RE, Boyles JK, Lee SH, Foss D, Mahley RW. Astrocytes synthesize apolipoprotein E and metabolize apolipoprotein E-containing lipoproteins. Biochim Biophys Acta. 1987;917:148–61.
5. Pitas RE, Boyles JK, Lee SH, Hui DY, Weisgraber KH. Lipoproteins and their receptors in the central nervous system: characterization of the lipoproteins in cerebrospinal fluid and identification of apolipoprotein B,E(LDL) receptors in the brain. J Biol Chem. 1987;262:14352–60.
6. Handelmann GE, Boyles JK, Weisgraber KH, Mahley RW, Pitas RE. Effects of apolipoprotein E, β-very low density lipoproteins, and cholesterol on the extension of neurites by rabbit dorsal root ganglion neurons in vitro. J Lipid Res. 1992;33:1677–88.
7. Müller HW, Gebicke-Härter PJ, Hangen DH, Shooter EM. A specific 37,000-dalton protein that accumulates in regenerating but not in nonregenerating mammalian nerves. Science. 1985;228:499–501.
8. Ignatius MJ, Gebicke-Härter PJ, Skene JHP, et al. Expression of apolipoprotein E during nerve degeneration and regeneration. Proc Natl Acad Sci USA. 1986;83:1125–9.
9. Boyles JK, Zoellner CD, Anderson LJ, et al. A role for apolipoprotein E, apolipoprotein A-I, and low density lipoprotein receptors in cholesterol transport during regeneration and remyelination of the rat sciatic nerve. J Clin Invest. 1989;83:1015–31.
10. Ignatius MJ, Shooter EM, Pitas RE, Mahley RW. Lipoprotein uptake by neuronal growth cones in vitro. Science. 1987;236:959–62.
11. Saunders AM, Strittmatter WJ, Schmechel D, et al. Association of apolipoprotein E allele ε4 with late-onset familial and sporadic Alzheimer's disease. Neurology. 1993;43:1467–72.
12. Corder EH, Saunders AM, Strittmatter WJ, et al. Gene dose of apolipoprotein E type 4 allele and the risk of Alzheimer's disease in late onset families. Science. 1993;261:921–3.
13. McKhann G, Drachman D, Folstein M, Katzman R, Price D, Stadlan EM. Clinical diagnosis of Alzheimer's disease: report of the NINCDS-ADRDA Work Group under the auspices of Department of Health and Human Services Task Force on Alzheimer's disease. Neurology. 1984;34:939–44.

14. Selkoe DJ. The molecular pathology of Alzheimer's disease. Neuron. 1991;6:487–98.
15. Crowther RA. Tau protein and paired helical filaments of Alzheimer's disease. Curr Opin Struct Biol. 1993;3:202–6.
16. Roses AD. The Alzheimer diseases. Curr Neurol. 1994;14:111–41.
17. Weisgraber KH, Roses AD, Strittmatter WJ. The role of apolipoprotein E in the nervous system. Curr Opin Lipidol. 1994;5:110–16.
18. Weisgraber KH, Pitas RE, Mahley RW. Lipoproteins, neurobiology, and Alzheimer's disease: structure and function of apolipoprotein E. Curr Opin Struct Biol. 1994;4:507–15.
19. Strittmatter WJ, Saunders AM, Schmechel D, et al. Apolipoprotein E: high avidity binding to β-amyloid and increased frequency of type 4 allele in late-onset familial Alzheimer disease. Proc Natl Acad Sci USA. 1993;90:1977–81.
20. Strittmatter WJ, Weisgraber KH, Huang DY, et al. Binding of human apolipoprotein E to synthetic amyloid β peptide: isoform-specific effects and implications for late-onset Alzheimer disease. Proc Natl Acad Sci USA. 1993;90:8098–102.
21. Sanan DA, Weisgraber KH, Russell SJ, et al. Apolipoprotein E associates with β amyloid peptide of Alzheimer's disease to form novel monofibrils. Isoform apoE4 associates more efficiently than apoE3. J Clin Invest. 1994;94:860–9.
22. Ma J, Yee A, Brewer HB Jr, Das S, Potter H. Amyloid-associated proteins α_1-antichymotrypsin and apolipoprotein E promote assembly of Alzheimer β-protein into filaments. Nature. 1994;372:92–4.
23. Strittmatter WJ, Weisgraber KH, Goedert M, et al. Hypothesis: microtubule instability and paired helical filament formation in the Alzheimer disease brain are related to apolipoprotein E genotype. Exp Neurol. 1994;125:163–71.
24. Nathan BP, Bellosta S, Sanan DA, Weisgraber KH, Mahley RW, Pitas RE. Differential effects of apolipoproteins E3 and E4 on neuronal growth *in vitro*. Science. 1994;264:850–2.
25. Nathan BP, Bellosta S, Mahley RW, Pitas RE. Apolipoprotein E3- and E4-induced differences in neurite outgrowth are associated with differences in the subcellular localization of apolipoprotein E. Soc Neurosci. 1994;20(Part 2):1033 (abstr.).

7

HDL metabolism and atherogenesis in genetically modified mice

N. MAEDA, S.H. ZHANG and R.L. REDDICK

INTRODUCTION

The genetics of atherosclerosis is complex, because many genes are involved and because the development of the disease is strongly influenced by environmental factors. Nevertheless, remarkable progress has been made in recent years through genetic analysis of human families and populations. In that way various candidate genes or candidate mutations have been identified that predispose individuals for premature atherosclerosis. Moving from strong correlations between mutations and phenotypes to proving that these factors are causative of atherosclerosis is, however, difficult to accomplish in the human system. For this purpose, mice generated by gene-targeting that carry precise changes in specific genes offer a unique approach to studying the role of discrete genetic factors in atherogenesis. It allows study not only of the effects in mice of candidate mutations found in humans, but also through genetic synthesis it allows study of the effects of various combinations of the mutations.

We and others have demonstrated that mice lacking apolipoprotein E (apoE) have elevated plasma cholesterol levels and develop atherosclerosis even on a regular low fat/low cholesterol diet[1,2]. The time-dependent progression of aortic lesions in these mutants parallels that observed in human patients[3,4]. Initial lesions are mainly of foam-cell deposits and are limited to the aortic sinus area in young mice (2–3 months old). By 5 months of age, developing atherosclerotic lesions are composed of foam-cell deposits, admixed smooth muscle cells and cholesterol crystals. In mice at 8–9 months of age the lesions contain fibrous caps, cholesterol clefts and calcification, and are widely distributed throughout the arterial tree. The rapid and predictable formation of atherosclerotic plaques in the mutants makes them valuable for studying the effects on lesion formation of adding other genetic and environmental factors.

In the present work we have used this system to test whether increased or decreased amounts of plasma apolipoprotein A-I (apoA-I) influence the development of atherosclerosis in the apoE-deficient mice. ApoA-I is the major protein component of HDL particles, and a correlation between decreased plasma levels of apoA-I and an elevated risk of coronary heart diseases has been well established in humans[5]. However, in some individuals with apoA-I deficiency, relatively mild or no coronary heart disease has been observed[6]. Mouse models should provide insights into the role of apoA-I and HDL in atherogenesis.

EFFECT OF THE TRANSGENIC HUMAN apoA-I GENE ON apoE-DEFICIENT MICE

Rubin et al.[7] have shown that the human apoA-I expressed in mice increases HDL cholesterol levels and protects mice from dietary-induced atherosclerosis. In collaboration with Dr Rubin and his associates we have crossed mice deficient in apoE with mice expressing the human apoA-I transgene in order to investigate whether elevated levels of apoA-I can protect mice from the atherosclerosis caused by the lack of apoE.

ApoE-deficient mice expressing the human apoA-I transgene (hAIt:E–/–) had a 2–3-fold increase in HDL levels compared to apoE-deficient mice (E–/–), but no change in non-HDL cholesterol. We found that the mean lesion size of 12-week-old hAIt:E–/– mice was 6-fold less than that in E–/– mice (Fig. 1). Of 22 hAIt:E–/– mice, 16 had no lesions or extremely small lesions, while all E–/– had lesions larger than 1000 μm^2. These data clearly show that elevated levels of apoA-I and HDL can significantly decelerate the development of atherosclerosis caused by the lack of apoE[8]. The same observation has independently been made by Plump et al.[9].

MICE LACKING APOLIPOPROTEIN A-I

In order to understand the role of decreased levels of apoA-I in lipid metabolism and atherogenesis, we have used gene-targeting to generate

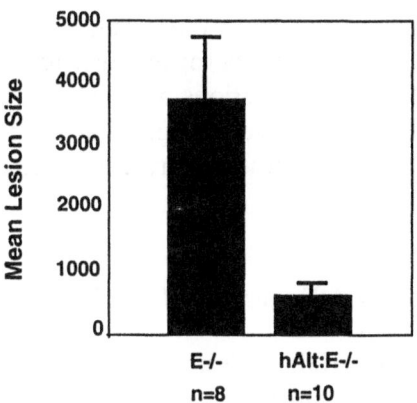

Fig. 1. Mean atherosclerotic lesion area per section (μm^2). Proximal aortas of animals were sectioned and the area of lesions were examined[8]. $p < 0.0001$ between two groups by Student's t-test

mice lacking apoA-I[10]. Total cholesterol in the homozygous mutants is approximately one-third that of their normal litter-mates. HDL cholesterol is reduced to an even greater extent (to 17% of normal). The homozygotes are grossly deficient in α-migrating lipoprotein particles. Thus the lipoprotein profiles of the mutant mice lacking apoA-I closely parallel those seen in human apoA-I deficiences. With such low HDL cholesterol levels we expected that the mutant mice would be prone to develop atherosclerosis; however, we have observed no sign of spontaneous atherosclerosis in mice lacking apoA-I. The proximal aortas were clean at 2 years of age in apoAI–/– mice that had been maintained on regular mouse chow[11].

We reasoned that a low level of HDL cholesterol in these mice was not in itself sufficient to cause atherosclerosis. We therefore tested whether feeding the mutant mice a high fat/high cholesterol diet could alter the development of lesions. Feeding the atherogenic diet to the apoAI–/– mutant mice increased their plasma cholesterol levels only by about 20 mg/dl, while levels in normal litter-mates increased by 60 mg/dl. This resistance of the apoA-I-deficient mice to a dietary increase of steady-state plasma cholesterol levels is somewhat surprising. It suggests that apoA-I may be necessary for the production of chylomicrons and/or VLDL, or that remnants of these particles may be cleaved more readily if apoA-I is lacking. Further detailed studies to investigate these possibilities are warranted.

We observed small fat deposits in the aorta, a sign of early athero-sclerotic lesions, in mice fed the atherogenic diet for 20 weeks, but the occurrence or extent of the depositions was not related to the apoA-I genotype. Taken together, our results imply that a simple reduction of apoA-I does not by itself cause atherosclerosis in mice even on high fat/ high cholesterol diet[11].

EFFECT OF THE LACK OF apoA-I ON apoE-DEFICIENT MICE

The levels of apoA-I and HDL cholesterol may be of importance when an individual has an increase in apoB-containing (atherogenic) particles. We took advantage of the relative ease of combining genetic factors in mice by crossbreeding to investigate the effect of reduced apoA-I in animals that lack apoE. By crossing mice lacking apoA-I and mice lacking apoE, doubly homozygous mutants were obtained at close to expected frequency.

The total plasma cholesterol in the double homozygotes (AI–/–:E–/–) is lower than apoE–/– mice (Fig. 2). HDL cholesterol levels are also significantly lower in double homozygotes than in apoE–/– mice. Total cholesterol levels as well as HDL cholesterol levels, are reduced in mice heterozygous for apoA-I mutation (AI+/–:E–/–). Thus the levels of non-HDL as well as HDL cholesterol directly correlate with apoA-I production in apoE–/– mice.

Our preliminary data suggest that the double homozygotes develop lesions earlier; the lesions in AI–/–:E–/– mice between 12 and 20 weeks old were about twice as large as in age-matched apoE–/– mice. On the other hand, the lesion sizes in 36-week-old AI–/–:E–/– mice were not different from those of apoE-deficient mice. The results so far suggest that lack of apoA-I may increase the initiation of atherosclerosis when apoE is also missing, but the mature lesions seen in older doubly mutant mice are not different in size from the lesions developed in mice lacking only apoE. Obviously these studies are at an early stage, and further detailed investigations are necessary.

CONCLUSION

A strength of using mice as an experimental system is the relative ease of combining genetic factors by crossbreeding. Mice completely lacking

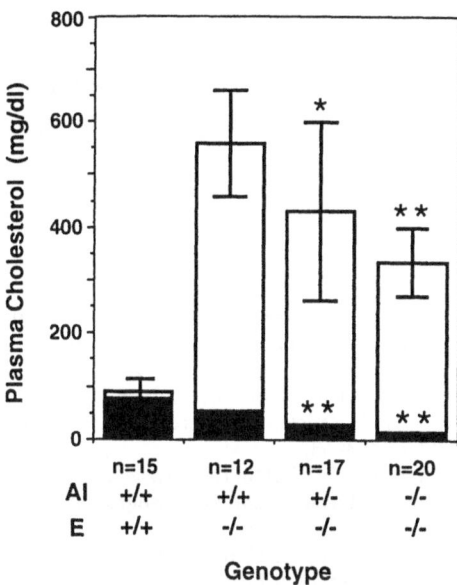

Fig. 2. Effect of reduced apoA-I on plasma cholesterol levels in apoE-deficient mice. Plasma total cholesterol levels of animals fasted overnight were measured as described[1]. Open boxes indicate total cholesterol with standard deviations. Portions of HDL cholesterol are shown by black boxes. Student's t-test was used to determine statistical significance (*$p < 0.01$; **$p < 0.0001$ against AI+/+:E−/− mice)

apoE predictably develop, on a regular mouse chow diet, atherosclerotic lesions with a complexity similar to that described in humans. Increasing the production of human apoA-I in mice lacking apoE reduces the lesion sizes, demonstrating the clear protective effect of apoA-I. On the other hand, mice lacking apoA-I do not develop atherosclerosis even on high fat/high cholesterol diet, implying that a simple lack of apoA-I by itself is not a cause of atherosclerosis in mice. The effects of reduced apoA-I production on the development of atherosclerosis in apoE-deficient mice may be subtle. Preliminary observations suggest that lack of apoA-I accelerates the initial development of lesions, but does not affect their eventual maturation. These examples serve to illustrate the ways in which genetically modified mice can be used to dissect the role of discrete genetic factors in atherogenesis.

Acknowledgements

The authors thank Lara Kester and Mynda Peyton for mouse colony maintenance and technical help. This work was supported by a NIH grant HL42630.

References

1. Zhang SH, Reddick RL, Piedrahita JA, Maeda N. Spontaneous hyper-cholesterolemia and arterial lesions in mice lacking apolipoprotein E. Science. 1992;258:468–71.
2. Plump AS, Smith JD, Hayet T, et al. Severe hypercholesterolemia and athero-sclerosis in apolipoprotein E-deficient mice created by homologous recombination in ES cells. Cell. 1992;71:343–53.
3. Reddick RL, Zhang SH, Maeda N. Atherosclerosis in mice lacking apolipoprotein E: evaluation of lesional development and progression. Arterioscler Thromb. 1994;14:141–7.
4. Nakashima Y, Plump AS, Raines EW, Breslow JL, Ross R. ApoE deficient mice develop lesions of all phases of atherosclerosis throughout the arterial tract. Arterioscler Thromb. 1994;14:133–40.
5. Maciejko JJ, Holmes DR, Kottke BA, Zinmeister AR, Dinh DM, Mao SJT. Apolipoprotein A-I as a marker of angiographically assessed coronary-artery disease. N Engl J Med. 1983;309:385–9.
6. Assmann G, von Eckardstein A, Funke H. High density lipoproteins, reverse transport of cholesterol and coronary artery disease: insights from mutations. Circulation. 1993;87(Suppl. III):III28–34.
7. Rubin EM, Krauss RM, Spangler EA, Verstuyft JG, Clift SM. Inhibition of early atherogenesis in transgenic mice by human apolipoprotein AI. Nature. 1991;353:265–7.
8. Paszty C, Maeda N, Verstuyft J, Rubin EM. Apolipoprotein AI transgene corrects apolipoprotein E deficiency-induced atherosclerosis in mice. J Clin Invest. 1994;94:899–903.
9. Plump AS, Scott CJ, Breslow JL. Human apolipoprotein A-I gene expression increases high density lipoprotein and suppresses atherosclerosis in the apolipo-protein E-deficient mouse. Proc Natl Acad Sci USA. 1994;91:9607–11.
10. Williamson R, Lee D, Hagaman J, Maeda N. Marked reduction of high density lipoprotein cholesterol in mice genetically modified to lack apolipoprotein A-I. Proc Natl Acad Sci USA. 1992;89:7134–8.
11. Li H, Reddick RL, Maeda N. Lack of apoA-I is not associated with increased susceptibility to atherosclerosis in mice. Arterioscler Thromb. 1993;13:1814–20.

8

Gene therapy for the genetic dyslipoproteinaemias

**H.B. BREWER, Jr, D.R. BROWN, V.S. KASHYAP,
D. APPLEBAUM-BOWDEN, J.M. HOEG, N. MAEDA and
S. SANTAMARINA-FOJO**

INTRODUCTION

Over the past two decades the roles of apolipoproteins, enzymes, lipoprotein receptors, and transfer proteins in lipoprotein metabolism have been elucidated. This new information provides a conceptual framework for understanding lipoprotein metabolism in normal subjects and patients with the genetic dyslipoproteinaemias. Schematic overviews of our current concepts of lipoprotein metabolism are illustrated in Figs. 1 and 2.

The human plasma lipoproteins can be conceptually separated into two separate pathways. One pathway involves the intravascular metabolic cascade of the apoB-containing lipoproteins (chylomicrons, very low density lipoproteins (VLDL), intermediate density lipoproteins (IDL), and low density lipoproteins (LDL) and the second pathway includes high density lipoproteins (HDL), the other major plasma lipoprotein.

OVERVIEW OF LIPOPROTEIN METABOLISM

The metabolism of the plasma lipoproteins containing the B apolipoproteins, apoB-48 and apoB-100, consists of two separate pathways[1-4]. The first apoB pathway involves the stepwise delipidation of triglyceride-rich chylomicron particles containing apoB-48 which transport dietary cholesterol and triglycerides from the intestine to peripheral tissues and ultimately to the liver. Following secretion, chylomicrons

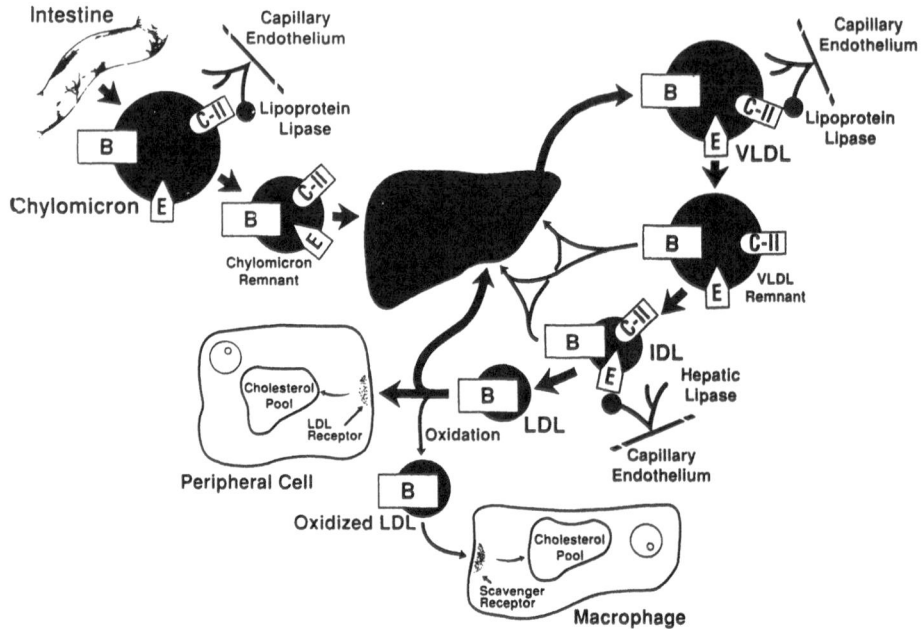

Fig. 1. Schematic overview of the major metabolic pathways for the metabolism of the apoB-containing lipoproteins including chylomicrons, VLDL, IDL, and LDL. The intestinal apoB pathway involves the stepwise delipidation of triglyceride-rich chylomicrons by lipoprotein lipase and its cofactor apoC-II, resulting in the formation of chylomicron remnant particles with an initial hydrated density of VLDL and finally IDL. In the hepatic apoB metabolic pathway, triglyceride-rich VLDL are converted to VLDL remnants, IDL and finally LDL. VLDL remnants and IDL may be removed from the plasma following interaction with the remnant and LDL receptors. The end-product of the VLDL cascade, LDL interact with LDL receptors which initiate receptor-mediated cellular uptake and degradation. LDL may also undergo oxidation with the formation of oxidized LDL which is taken up by the macrophage via the scavenger receptor and contributes to the development of the atherosclerotic lesion (see text for further details).

acquire two apolipoproteins, apoE and apoC-II, present on HDL. ApoC-II activates the endothelium-bound lipoprotein lipase (LPL) enzyme which results in triglyceride hydrolysis and intravascular remodelling with conversion of the triglyceride-rich chylomicrons to small chylomicron remnants with a hydrated density of initially VLDL and then IDL. Concomitant with the hydrolysis of triglycerides, apolipoproteins as well as lipid constituents are transferred from chylomicrons to HDL.

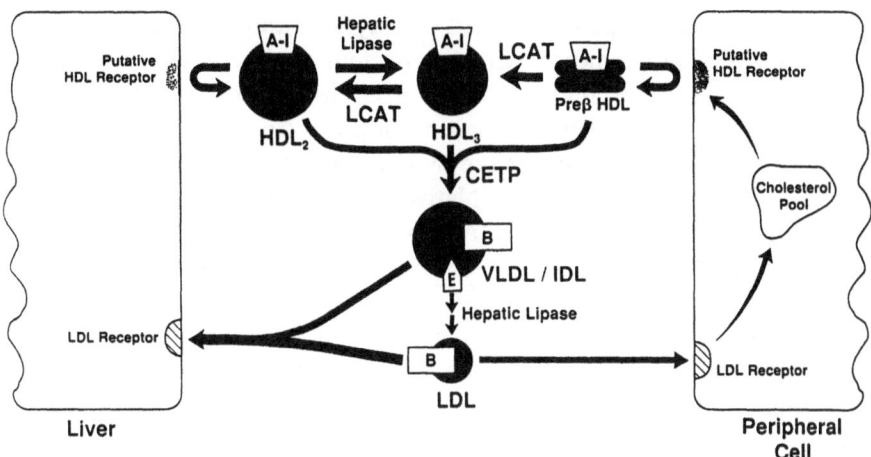

Fig. 2. Schematic overview of HDL and reverse cholesterol transport. Excess cellular cholesterol is removed by nascent preβ-HDL following interaction with a putative HDL receptor. Cholesterol is converted to cholesteryl esters by LCAT and the nascent HDL is converted to particles with a hydrated density of HDL_3 and then HDL_2. Cholesteryl esters are transferred directly either to the liver or to VLDL-IDL-LDL by CETP. The apoB-containing lipoprotein particles play an important role in reverse cholesterol transport by transporting the cholesteryl esters derived from HDL back to the liver (see text for additional details).

The second apoB pathway involves triglyceride-rich VLDL containing apoB-100 secreted by the liver. ApoC-II and apoE dissociate from HDL and reassociate with the hepatogenous triglyceride-rich VLDL secreted from the liver. ApoC-II activates LPL as outlined above, and VLDL are serially converted to VLDL remnants, IDL, and finally LDL. Hepatic lipase, a second lipolytic enzyme, and apoE have been proposed to be required for the efficient conversion of IDL to LDL. During the metabolic conversion of VLDL to LDL approximately 50% of VLDL remnants and IDL are removed from the plasma by the liver.

Remnants of both the chylomicron and VLDL pathways have been proposed to be removed from the plasma primarily by the interaction of apoE as well as apoB-100 with the hepatic remnant and LDL receptors, respectively[5–8].

LDL, the final lipoprotein in the VLDL cascade, contains virtually only apoB-100, and interacts primarily with the LDL receptor present on the plasma membrane of the liver (Fig. 1). In addition, LDL interact with the LDL receptor on peripheral cells including adrenal, fibroblasts and smooth muscle cells[6,7]. The interaction of LDL with the LDL receptor initiates receptor-mediated endocytosis and transport of LDL to intracellular lysosomes, where the protein moiety is degraded and cholesteryl esters are hydrolysed to free cholesterol, which is then transferred to the intracellular cholesterol pool. An additional pathway for LDL metabolism is the uptake by macrophages with the formation of foam cells in the arterial wall. Native LDL is not readily taken up by macrophages. However, oxidative modification of LDL results in markedly enhanced LDL uptake by the scavenger receptor on macrophages with foam cell formation[9-12]. Oxidative modifications of LDL were observed following *in-vitro* incubation with endothelial cells, smooth muscle cells, and macrophages, or following modification with malondialdehyde. Recent studies have indicated that oxidized lipids within LDL may play an important role in the pathophysiology of the atherosclerotic lesion by stimulating the secretion of cytokines and other factors which modulate endothelial cell function, as well as facilitating the recruitment of plasma monocytes into the vessel wall[13]. Based on current data it has been proposed that oxidative modification of LDL may be a prerequisite for the macrophage uptake of LDL, foam-cell formation, and the development of the atherosclerotic lesion.

The major role of HDL in lipoprotein metabolism is to transport cholesterol from peripheral tissues back to the liver, where it is removed from the body following conversion to bile acids or as biliary cholesterol. This hypothetical process, designated reverse cholesterol transport[14,15], is shown schematically in Fig. 2. Nascent HDL, composed primarily of apoA-I phospholipid discs, are secreted from both the human intestine and liver. Nascent HDL acquire excess cholesterol from tissues, and the enzyme lecithin cholesterol acyltransferase (LCAT) catalyses the esterification of plasma lipoprotein cholesterol to cholesteryl esters. With the formation of cholesteryl esters the nascent HDL are converted to spherical lipoproteins with a hydrated density of HDL_3. HDL_3 are converted to the larger HDL_2 by the acquisition of apolipoproteins and lipids released during the stepwise delipidation and remodelling of the triglyceride-rich chylomicrons and VLDL, as well as by the esterification of the cholesterol removed from peripheral tissues. HDL is proposed to transfer the cholesterol removed from the peripheral tissues to the liver. HDL_2 are converted back to HDL_3 by hepatic lipase through the removal of phospholipids and triglycerides, and the generation of nascent apoA-I HDL[1,14-19]. The cycle of uptake of cholesterol from peripheral tissues, transport of the cholesterol to the liver, and regeneration of nascent HDL is repeated as cholesterol is transported from the periphery to the liver. An additional pathway for transport of cholesterol to the liver is the transfer of cholesteryl esters in HDL to VLDL-IDL-LDL by the cholesterol ester transfer protein (CETP), which delivers cholesterol to the liver by the apoB-containing lipoproteins[20]. In this proposed model of reverse cholesterol transport the removal of cholesterol from the peripheral cell involves the interaction of HDL with a putative HDL receptor on peripheral cells and the liver. The precise nature of the specific HDL receptor involved in the transport of cholesterol from peripheral cells back to the liver, where it can be excreted from the body, remains to be definitively established.

CLASSIFICATION OF THE MOLECULAR DEFECTS IN THE GENETIC DYSLIPOPROTEINAEMIAS

The major molecular defects in the genetic dyslipoproteinaemias are due to defects either in apolipoproteins, enzymes, or lipoprotein receptors. The elucidation of the molecular defects in patients resulting in the genetic dyslipoproteinaemias provides the opportunity for ultimate definitive correction of these gene defects by somatic gene therapy. The availability of animal models with selective defects in lipoprotein metabolism, as well as mice models with selective 'gene knockouts' developed by homologous recombination, permits the evaluation of currently available vectors for gene replacement. This report will summarize the available information on the initial gene therapy studies in humans and the results on three animal models we have chosen to illustrate gene replacement of a lipoprotein receptor, apolipoprotein, and a lipolytic enzyme.

GENE THERAPY FOR THE GENETIC DYSLIPOPROTEINAEMIAS

Gene therapy for genetic defects in lipoprotein receptors

LDL receptor

Initial studies on the correction of the LDL receptor defect in patients with familial hypercholesterolaemia have been performed utilizing an

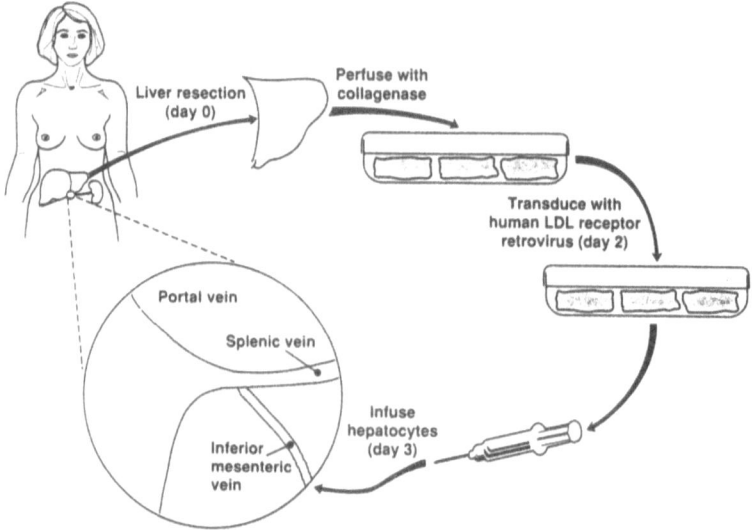

Fig. 3. Strategy for gene therapy of the LDL receptor defect in patients with familial hypercholesterolaemia using an *ex-vivo* approach with autologous hepatocytes corrected with recombinant retrovirus carrying the LDL receptor (adapted from ref. 21)

ex-vivo approach with autologous hepatocytes corrected with recombinant retroviruses carrying the LDL receptor. The first patient in this series of studies was a 28-year-old French Canadian woman who had suffered a myocardial infarction at the age of 16 and had coronary artery bypass surgery at the age of 26[21]. The patient was receptor-defective with a missense mutation ($Trp_{66}Gly$) in the LDL receptor. Pretreatment plasma lipid values included a total cholesterol level of 545 mg/dl, LDL of 482 mg/dl, and an HDL of 43 mg/dl. Cardiac catheterization revealed significant coronary atherosclerosis.

A schematic overview of the strategy of the *ex-vivo* gene therapy for familial hypercholesterolaemia reported by Wilson and colleagues is shown in Fig. 3[21]. The left lateral segment of the liver is removed, perfused with collagenase to release the hepatocytes, and hepatocytes were cultured *in vitro*. The LDL receptor defect in the cultured hepatocytes was corrected using a recombinant retrovirus expressing the LDL receptor. The genetically corrected transduced hepatocytes were harvested and infused back into the patient via a catheter in the inferior mesenteric vein.

Analysis by *in-situ* hybridization of liver tissue obtained by percutaneous biopsy 4 months after gene therapy was positive, indicating successful transgene expression in the liver[21]. The plasma LDL cholesterol decreased 17%, HDL cholesterol increased 8%, and the LDL/HDL ratio decreased from 11 ± 0.04 to 7.9 ± 0.9. Following the initiation of lovastatin drug therapy LDL cholesterol decreased 14%, and the LDL/HDL ratio decreased from 7.9 ± 0.9 to 6.6 ± 0.6. The combined results from this initial gene therapy trial established that primary hepatocytes obtained from partial hepatectomy could be corrected *in vitro*. The genetically corrected hepatocytes could be effectively infused back into the patient for seeding of the transduced cells in the liver[21]. The major limitation of this *ex-vivo* gene therapy approach is the small number of cells that can be safely and effectively delivered back to the patient, which does not appear to be sufficient to totally correct the plasma lipoprotein profile. Thus, the *ex-vivo* approach may not be the best form of gene therapy for these patients, since only partial correction of the defect can be achieved.

The limitations of the *ex-vivo* approach for the total correction of the LDL receptor defect in familial hypercholesterolaemia have led to the initiation of other methods for gene delivery. We have evaluated the potential role of adenovirus gene therapy in the rabbit animal model for the LDL receptor defect. The LDL receptor-deficient rabbit has a plasma cholesterol of 400–600 mg/dl, triglycerides of 60–120 mg/dl, and HDL cholesterol of 30–42 mg/dl[22-25]. The adenovirus vector utilized in these studies had the E1a and E1b regions deleted and replaced with a cDNA cassette containing the LDL receptor, as well as the CMV immediate-early enhancer and promoter, SV40 RNA splicing signals and the SV40 transcription termination and polyadenylation signal[26-29]. Recombinant LDL receptor-adenovirus (5×10^{10} pfu) was injected intravenously into LDL receptor-deficient rabbits. Total cholesterol levels were reduced to up to 56% of pretreatment values, reaching a maximal decrease at days 2–4 with gradual return to baseline at 2–3 weeks. ApoA-I levels increased 85% above pretreatment levels with a maximum value at day 10. These combined results indicate that the adenovirus may represent an effective approach to the treatment of LDL receptor deficiency. In addition the reciprocal changes in the plasma cholesterol and apoA-I illustrate the metabolic interrelationship of LDL and HDL.

Gene therapy for genetic defects in plasma apolipoproteins

Apolipoprotein E

ApoE plays a key role in lipoprotein metabolism, as outlined above, by facilitating the cellular uptake of remnants of triglyceride-rich chylomicrons and VLDL[2,30] by serving as a ligand on lipoprotein particles for the LDL receptor and LRP, the putative remnant receptor[31-36]. The important role that apoE plays in lipoprotein transport has been established in part by identification of patients with apoE deficiency[37-41] or, more commonly, patients with a structural defect in apoE which results in decreased affinity for plasma lipoprotein receptors[42-45]. A defect in the function of apoE leads to delayed plasma clearance of remnants of triglyceride-rich lipoproteins and the development of dysbetalipoproteinaemia or type III hyperlipoproteinaemia. Kindreds with apoE deficiency and type III hyperlipoproteinaemia have been extensively studied and are characterized by elevated plasma levels of cholesterol, triglycerides, cholesterol-rich remnants of chylomicrons and VLDL, as well as by xanthomas and premature cardiovascular disease[37-41].

A mouse model for apoE deficiency has been developed using homologous recombination with apoE targeted gene disruption in embryonic stem cells[46]. The apoE 'knockout' mice develop marked hypercholesterolaemia with total cholesterol levels 5–6-fold greater than control mice[47-48]. These apoE-deficient mice have a dramatic shift in plasma lipoproteins from HDL, the major lipoprotein in control mice, to cholesterol-enriched remnants of chylomicrons and VLDL. Of particular interest in the apoE-deficient mice is the development of spontaneous atherosclerosis on a normal chow diet[48-49]. The apoE-deficient mouse represents a unique model to study gene replacement of a plasma apolipoprotein for correction of a genetic dyslipoproteinaemia.

The correction of the apoE deficiency in the apoE-deficient animal model presents several interesting challenges. For apoE to function in facilitating the clearance of lipoprotein remnants, gene replacement must be followed by synthesis and secretion of the apolipoprotein in a pathway which will permit it to become associated with both hepatic endothelial proteoglycans and plasma lipoproteins. In addition, to achieve physiological replacement with apoE, the transgene must be

Table 1. Plasma lipids and lipoproteins (mg/dl) in control mice, apoE-deficient mice, and apoE-deficient mice following recombinant apoE adenovirus infusion

	TC	TG	PL	CE	FC
Controls (*n*=15)	103±13	76±17	185±17	77±10	26±4
ApoE-deficient (*n*=15)	644±149	111±74	341±82	420±121	223±49
Adv-Rx-ApoE-deficient (*n*=7)	103±18	97±32	194±34	52±10	52±12

expressed in the mg/dl level in plasma which has not been readily achieved in previous gene replacement studies.

The plasma lipids and lipoproteins present in the apoE-deficient and control C57 black mice are summarized in Table 1. When compared to control mice the apoE-deficient mice were markedly hyperlipidaemic with plasma total cholesterol, cholesteryl ester and free cholesterol levels approximately 6-fold greater than control mice, and plasma triglycerides and phospholipids 2-fold greater. Furthermore, HDL is reduced to one-third of the normal levels.

We have successfully corrected the apoE deficiency in the apoE 'knockout' mice utilizing an adenovirus vector containing the human apoE cDNA. The apoE cDNA was subcloned into a shuttle vector (pAd12apoE) containing a CMV enhancer and promoter elements, a SV40 polyadenylation signal, and the E1 region of the human adenovirus (Ad5). The recombinant virus was propagated in 293 cells and purified by caesium chloride density ultracentrifugation.

Following apoE-adenovirus infusion the hypercholesterolaemia, as well as the lipoprotein profile, were normalized for a period of up to 3 weeks with plasma apoE levels ranging from a physiological level of 3–4 mg/dl to 650 mg/dl. The lipoprotein profiles of the apoE-deficient mice after apoE adenovirus gene therapy are summarized in Table 1. Successful replacement of apoE in apoE-deficient mice demonstrates the feasibility of gene therapy in human apolipoprotein deficiencies[56].

Gene therapy for genetic defects in enzymes

Hepatic lipase

Hepatic lipase plays a key role in lipoprotein metabolism in the conversion of IDL to LDL and HDL_2 to HDL_3. Patients with a deficiency of hepatic lipase have a type III-like lipoprotein phenotype with increased plasma levels of cholesterol, triglycerides, and IDL[50-55]. In addition these kindreds show an increased plasma level of HDL_2. Clinically these patients may have palmar and tuberous xanthomas, as well as an increased risk of premature cardiovascular disease. A hepatic lipase-deficient mouse model has been developed by gene disruption using homologous recombination[57]. The lipoprotein profile of the hepatic lipase-deficient mouse model is summarized in Table 2. When compared to controls, hepatic lipase-deficient animals have approximately 2-fold increased plasma levels of total cholesterol, phospholipids, cholesteryl esters, and HDL cholesterol.

Table 2. Plasma lipids and lipoproteins (mg/dl) in control mice, hepatic lipase (HL)-deficient mice, and hepatic lipase-deficient mice following recombinant hepatic lipase adenovirus infusion

	TC	TG	PL	CE	HDL-C
Controls (n=13)	101 ± 2	63 ± 2	211 ± 4	66 ± 2	78 ± 3
HL deficiency (n=7)	176 ± 9	58 ± 4	314 ± 12	122 ± 9	129 ± 9
Adv-Rx HL deficiency (n=5)	94 ± 10	51 ± 5	207 ± 16	35 ± 12	62 ± 8

The successful replacement of the hepatic lipase gene in the hepatic lipase-deficient mice using the adenovirus vector system has several requirements. The human hepatic lipase gene must be delivered to the liver, hepatic lipase must be synthesized as well as undergo post-translational processing and secretion from the cell, followed by binding of the active enzyme to the endothelial glycosaminoglycans, where it must be effective in hydrolysing plasma lipoprotein triglycerides and phospholipids.

The complete correction of the lipoprotein profile in the hepatic lipase-deficient mouse has been achieved using the human cDNA recombinant adenovirus under the control of the CMV promoter and enhancer, an SV40 splice donor and acceptor, as well as an SV40 polyadenylation signal sequence. Plasma hepatic lipase mass by immunoblot analysis and enzymic activity were used to quantitate gene replacement in the hepatic lipase-deficient mouse after hepatic lipase adenovirus infusion. Following intravenous injection of 10^9 pfu of hepatic lipase–adenovirus constructs, the post-heparin plasma hepatic lipase activity maximally increased 100 times over pretreatment values. Hepatic lipase activity reached a maximum at days 4–6 and could be detected in 50% of the animals at 30 days. The plasma lipoprotein profile in hepatic lipase-deficient mice following hepatic lipase adenovirus infusion is summarized in Table 2. The post-treatment FPLC profile was normalized with total cholesterol, phospholipids, and cholesteryl esters decreased by 80% and triglycerides reduced by approximately 50%. Post-heparin injection revealed that >90% of the human hepatic lipase enzyme was bound to the capillary endothelium, establishing that the enzyme was transported from the hepatocyte to the capillary endothelium where it bound to the glycosaminoglycans and was enzymically active[58].

SUMMARY

The combined studies reported here detail the initial approaches that have been used for gene therapy for familial hypercholesterolaemia in human and animal models for the genetic dyslipoproteinaemias. Limited success has been achieved using the *ex-vivo* hepatic retroviral-mediated approach to the correction of the genetic defect in patients with familial hypercholesterolaemia. The present studies indicate that genetic defects in the genetic dyslipoproteinaemias can be effectively corrected using adenovirus vectors. The complete correction of the apoE and hepatic lipase deficiencies in the knockout mice models established that it will be possible to correct genetic defects due to both apolipoproteins and lipolytic enzymes. In humans the ultimate effective correction of these genetic defects now awaits the development of additional vector systems that will be both safe and provide long-term expression of transgenes in patients with genetic dyslipoproteinaemias.

References

1. Brewer HB, Jr, Gregg RE, Hoeg JM, Fojo SS. Apolipoproteins and lipoproteins in human plasma: an overview. Clin Chem. 1988;34:4–8.
2. Brewer HB, Jr, Gregg RE, Hoeg JM. Apolipoproteins, lipoproteins, and atherosclerosis. In: Braunwald E, editor. Heart disease: a textbook of cardiovascular medicine. New York: W.B. Saunders; 1989:121–44.
3. Vega GL, Denke MA, Grundy SM. Metabolic basis of primary hypercholesterolaemia. Circulation. 1991;84:118–28.
4. Schaefer EJ. Diagnosis and management of lipoprotein disorders. In: Rifkind BM, editor. Drug treatment of hyperlipidemia. New York: Marcel Dekker; 1991:17–52.
5. Davignon J, Gregg RE, Sing CF. Apolipoproteins E polymorphism and atherosclerosis. Arteriosclerosis. 1988;8:1–21.
6. Goldstein JL, Brown MS. The LDL receptor locus and the genetics of familial hypercholesterolemia. Annu Rev Genet. 1979;13:259–89.
7. Goldstein JL, Brown MS, Anderson RG, Russell DW, Schneider WJ. Receptor-mediated endocytosis: concepts emerging from the LDL receptor system. Annu Rev Cell Biol. 1985;1:1–39.
8. Gregg RE, Brewer HB, Jr. The role of apolipoproteins E and lipoprotein receptors in modulating the *in vivo* metabolism of apolipoproteins B-containing lipoproteins in humans. Clin Chem. 1988;34:28–32.
9. Steinberg D. Lipoproteins and atherosclerosis. A look back and a look ahead. Arteriosclerosis. 1983;3:283–301.
10. Steinberg D. Antioxidants and atherosclerosis: a current assessment. Circulation. 1991;84:1420–5.
11. Van Lenten BJ, Fogelman AM. Processing of lipoproteins in human monocyte-macrophages. J Lipid Res. 1990;31:1455–66.
12. Haberland ME, Fogelman AM. The role of altered lipoproteins in the pathogenesis of atherosclerosis. Am Heart J. 1987;113:573–7.
13. Navab M, Hama SY, Nguyen TB, Fogelman AM. Monocyte adhesion and transmigration in atherosclerosis. Coronary Artery Dis. 1994;5:198–204.
14. Glomset JA, Janssen ET, Kennedy R, Dobbins J. Role of plasma lecithin:cholesterol acyltransferase in the metabolism of high density lipoproteins. J Lipid Res. 1966;7:638–48.
15. Glomset JA. The plasma lecithin:cholesterol acyltransferase reaction. J Lipid Res. 1968;9:155–67.
16. Eisenberg S. High density lipoprotein metabolism. J Lipid Res. 1984;25: 1017–58.
17. Radar DJ, Castro G, Zech LA, Fruchart JC, Brewer HB, Jr. *In vivo* metabolism of apolipoproteins A-I on high density lipoprotein particles LpA-I and LpA-I, A-II. J Lipid Res. 1991;32:1849–59.
18. Brinton EA, Eisenberg S, Breslow JL. Human HDL cholesterol levels are determined by apoA-I fractional catabolic rate, which correlates inversely with estimates of HDL particle size: effects of gender, hepatic and lipoprotein lipases, triglyceride and insulin levels, and body fat distribution. Arterioscler Thromb. 1994;14:707–20.
19. Grundy SM. Multifactorial etiology of hypercholesterolemia: implications for prevention of coronary heart disease. Arterioscler Thromb. 1991;11: 1619–35.
20. Tall AR. Plasma cholesteryl ester transfer protein. J Lipid Res. 1993;34: 1255–74.
21. Grossman M, Raper SE, Kozarsky K, et al. Successful *ex-vivo* gene therapy directed to liver in a patient with familial hypercholesterolaemia. Nature Genet. 1994;6:335–41.

22. Watanabe Y. Serial inbreeding of rabbits with hereditary hyperlipidemia (WHHL-rabbit): incidence and development of atherosclerosis and xanthoma. Atherosclerosis. 1980;36:261–8.
23. Tanzawa K, Shimada Y, Kuroda M, Tsujita Y, Arai M, Watanabe H. WHHL-rabbit: a low density lipoprotein receptor-deficient animal model for familial hypercholesterolemia. FEBS Lett. 1980;118:81–4.
24. Buja LM, Kita T, Goldstein JL, Watanabe Y, Brown MS. Cellular pathology of progressive atherosclerosis in the WHHL rabbit: an animal model of familial hypercholesterolemia. Arteriosclerosis. 1983;3:87–101.
25. Yamamoto T, Bishop RW, Brown MS, Goldstein JL, Russell DW. Deletion in cysteine-rich region of LDL receptor impedes transport to cell surface in WHHL rabbit. Science. 1986;232:1230–7.
26. Chen C, Okayama H. High-efficiency transformation of mammalian cells by plasmid DNA. Mol Cell Biol. 1987;7:2745–52.
27. Graham FL, Smiley J, Russel WC, Nairn R. Characteristics of a human cell line transformed by DNA from human adenovirus type 5. J Gen Virol. 1977;36:59–72.
28. Harrison T, Graham F, Williams J. Host-range mutants of adenovirus type 5 defective for growth in HeLa cells. Virology. 1977;77:319–29.
29. Green M, Pina M. Biochemical studies on adenovirus multiplication: IV. Isolation, purification, and chemical analysis of adenovirus. Virology. 1963;20:199–207.
30. Mahley RW. Apolipoprotein E: cholesterol transport protein with expanding role in cell biology. Science. 1988;240:622–30.
31. Mahley RW, Innerarity TL, Weisgraber KH, et al. Cellular and molecular biology of lipoprotein metabolism: characterization of lipoprotein receptor–ligand interactions. Cold Spring Harbor Symp Quant Biol. 1986;51:821–8.
32. Nykjaer A, Bengtsson-Olivecrona G, Lookene A, et al. The α_2-macroglobulin receptor/low density lipoprotein receptor-related protein binds lipoprotein lipase and β-migrating very low density lipoprotein associated with the lipase. J Biol Chem. 1993;268:15048–55.
33. Mulder M, Lombardi P, Jansen H, Van Berkel TJC, Frants RR, Havekes LM. Low density lipoprotein receptor internalizes low density and very low density lipoproteins that are bound to heparan sulfate proteoglycans via lipoprotein lipase. J Biol Chem. 1993;268:9369–75.
34. Mahley RW, Ji ZS, Brecht WJ, Miranda RD, He D. Role of heparan sulfate proteoglycans and the LDL receptor-related protein in remnant lipoprotein metabolism. Ann NY Acad Sci. 1994;737:39–52.
35. Santamarina-Fojo S, Dugi K. Structure, function and role of lipoprotein lipase in lipoprotein metabolism. Curr Opin Lipidol. 1994;5:117–25.
36. Takahashi S, Kawarabayasi Y, Nakai T, Sakai J, Yamamoto T. Rabbit very low density lipoprotein receptor: a low density lipoprotein receptor-like protein with distinct ligand specificity. Proc Natl Acad Sci USA. 1992;89:9252–6.
37. Ghiselli G, Schaefer EJ, Gascon P, Brewer HB, Jr. Type III hyperlipoproteinemia associated with apolipoprotein E deficiency. Science. 1981;214:1239–41.
38. Schaefer EJ, Gregg RE, Ghiselli G, et al. Familial apolipoprotein E deficiency. J Clin Invest. 1986;78:1206–19.
39. Mabuchi H, Itoh H, Takeda M, et al. A young type III hyperlipoproteinemic patient associated with apolipoprotein E deficiency. Metabolism. 1989;38:115–19.
40. Kurosaka D, Teramoto T, Matsushima T, et al. Apolipoprotein E deficiency with a depressed mRNA of normal size. Atherosclerosis. 1991;88:15–20.

41. Lohse P, Brewer HB, III, Meng MS, Skarlatos SI, LaRosa JC, Brewer HB, Jr. Familial apolipoprotein E deficiency and type III hyperlipoproteinemia due to a premature stop codon in the apolipoprotein E gene. J Lipid Res. 1992;33:1583–90.
42. Zannis VI, Breslow JL. Characterization of a unique human apolipoprotein E variant associated with type III hyperlipoproteinemia. J Biol Chem. 1980;255: 1759–62.
43. Brewer HB, Jr, Zech LA, Gregg RA, Schwartz D, Schaefer EJ. Type III hyperlipoproteinemia: diagnosis, molecular defects, pathology, and treatment. Ann Intern Med. 1983;98:623–40.
44. Brewer HB, Jr, Santamarina-Fojo S, Hoeg JM. Disorders of lipoprotein metabolism. In: DeGroot LJ, Besser M, Jameson JL, et al. Endocrinology. Philadelphia: W.B. Saunders; 1995:2731–53.
45. Mahley RW, Rall SC, Jr. Type III hyperlipoproteinemia (dysbetalipoproteinemia): the role of apolipoprotein E in normal and abnormal lipoprotein metabolism. In: Scriver CR, Beaudet AL, Sly WS, et al. The metabolic and molecular bases of inherited disease. New York: McGraw-Hill; 1995:1953–80.
46. Thomas KR, Capecchi MR. Site-directed mutagenesis by gene targeting in mouse embryo-derived stem cells. Cell. 1987;51:503–12.
47. Piedrahita JA, Zhang SH, Hagaman JR, Oliver PM, Maeda N. Generation of mice carrying a mutant apolipoprotein E gene inactivated by gene targeting in embryonic stem cells. Proc Natl Acad Sci USA. 1992;89: 4471–5.
48. Plump AS, Smith JD, Hayek T, et al. Severe hypercholesterolemia and atherosclerosis in apolipoprotein E-deficient mice created by homologous recombination in ES cells. Cell. 1992;71:343–53.
49. Zhang SH, Reddick RL, Piedrahita JA, Maeda N. Spontaneous hypercholesterolemia and arterial lesions in mice lacking apolipoprotein E. Science. 1992;258:468–71.
50. Breckenridge WC, Little JA, Alaupovic P, et al. Lipoprotein abnormalities associated with a familial deficiency of hepatic lipase. Atherosclerosis. 1982;45:161–79.
51. Carlson LA, Holmquist L, Nilsson-Ehle P. Deficiency of hepatic lipase activity in post-heparin plasma in familial hyper-α-triglyceridemia. Acta Med Scand. 1986;219:435–47.
52. Auwerx JH, Marzetta CA, Hokanson JE, Brunzell JD. Large buoyant LDL-like particles in hepatic lipase deficiency. Arteriosclerosis. 1989;9: 319–25.
53. Auwerx JH, Babirak SP, Hokanson JE, et al. Coexistence of abnormalities of hepatic lipase and lipoprotein lipase in a large family. Am J Hum Genet. 1990;46:470–7.
54. Ikeda Y, Takagi A. Hypertriglyceridemia in a deficiency of lipoprotein lipase and hepatic lipase. Tanpakushitsu Kakusan Koso. 1988;33:783–90.
55. Connelly PW, Maguire GF, Lee M, Little JA. Plasma lipoproteins in familial hepatic lipase deficiency. Arteriosclerosis. 1990;10:40–8.
56. Homanics GE, de Silva HV, Osada J, et al. Mild dyslipidemia in mice following targeted inactivation of the hepatic lipase gene. J Biol Chem. 1995;270:2974–80.
57. Kashyap VS, Santamarina-Fojo S, Brown DR, et al. 1995, in press.
58. Applebaum-Bowden D, Kobayashi J, Brown D, et al. Gene replacement of a lipolytic enzyme in HL-deficient mice. Circulation. 1994;90:I-407.

Index

neurites, extension/branching, effects of
   apoE3/4 56–7
neurofibrillary tangles, Alzheimer's
   disease, and apoE 55
niacin 37–8
Niemann–Pick disease (type C) 43

ox-LDL
   and atherogenesis 35–6
   cytotoxicity 35
   and macrophage interaction 35
β-oxidation, peroxisomal/mitochondrial
   3-ketoacyl-CoA substrates 49–
   50

peripheral nerve injury, apoE levels 54
peroxisomes, and cholesterol
   biosynthesis 50
phosphatidylcholine (PC) transfer, and
   SCP2/SCPx 48
preβ$_1$-LpA-I, transfer to LDL 19
pregnenolone, biosynthesis pathways
   43–4

restriction fragment length
   polymorphisms (RFLPs), and
   CAD prediction 4

simvastatin 37–8
sterol carrier protein 2 (SCP2) 44–51
   7-DHC conversion to cholesterol 44,
   47
   α-β-tertiary fold 48
   α-helices, and nuclear Overhauser
   effects 48
   gene, exon 14 region, restriction
   nuclease map 50–1

phosphatidylcholine transfer 48
sterol/phospholipid transfer,
   structural basis 48–51
transcripts, alternative splicing/
   alternative transcription
   initiation 45
sterol carrier protein 2 (SCP2) thiolase
   50
sterol carrier protein 2 (SCP2)-ps1 45
sterol carrier protein 2 (SCP2)-ps2 45
sterol carrier protein x (SCPx) 45–51
   3-ketoacyl-CoA substrates, thiolytic
   cleavage 46–7
   α-helices, and nuclear Overhauser
   effects 48
   biological functions 46
   gene, exon 14 region, restriction
   nuclease map 50–1
   peroxisomal localization 46
   phosphatidylcholine transfer 48
   sterol/phospholipid transfer,
   structural basis 48–51
   transcripts, alternative splicing/
   alternative transcription
   initiation 45

Tangier disease 17, 20–1, 43
tau, interaction with apoE3/4 55
thiolases, SCPx 46–7

vitamins C/E, LDL oxidation inhibition
   35, 37–8
VLDL, conversion to LDL 68–9

Zellweger disease 43